P9-DIH-512

PRAISE FOR

THE COMPLETE LOW-FODMAP DIET

"IBS has been a daunting problem for patients and their physicians for years. We have seen many drugs and different dietary fads come and go. So, it is wonderful that Sue Shepherd and Peter Gibson have developed this solution for many patients with IBS: a diet based on sound scientific and physiological mechanisms. Combined with good medical care that includes testing for small intestinal bacterial overgrowth and fructose and lactose intolerance, the low-FODMAP diet can be individualized, liberalized, and tailored to each patient. This book also provides a great deal of information as to how the diet can be truly indulged in!"

—PETER H. R. GREEN, MD, Professor of Clinical Medicine and Director of the Celiac Disease Center at Columbia University

"The low-FODMAP diet has revolutionized my practice and has helped so many of my patients. If you suffer from irritable bowel syndrome and choosing food is a challenge, this splendid book is a must-have survival guide. Begin your journey back to good gut health by using food as medicine. Kudos to Drs. Shepherd and Gibson!"

—GERARD E. MULLIN, MD, Associate Professor of Medicine and Director of Integrative GI Nutrition Services at the Johns Hopkins University School of Medicine, and coauthor of *The Inside Tract*, http://thefoodmd.com

"For those with celiac disease who continue to have digestive issues, *The Complete Low-FODMAP Diet* is a must-read. Drs. Shepherd and Gibson do a tremendous job both in identifying the foods responsible for digestive distress and in offering a personalized approach to a balanced diet free from those triggers. With science-based information and easy-to-follow recipes, this book delivers the *why* and *how* that people are looking to know."

—ALICE BAST, President of the National Foundation for Celiac Awareness (NFCA)

"Drs. Shepherd and Gibson have truly created a complete reference guide about the low-FODMAP diet. The book offers evidence that supports the use of the low-FODMAP diet to manage digestive symptoms, especially IBS. The authors walk you through precise diets, recipes, and menus to put the diet into practice. The recipes are easy to follow and the illustrations are quite breathtaking. I strongly recommend this book for all IBS sufferers."

—JEFFREY D. ROBERTS, Founder of IBS Self Help and Support Group, www.ibsgroup.com

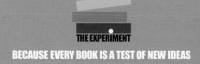

THE EXPERIMENT

BECAUSE EVERY BOOK IS A TEST OF NEW IDEAS

ALSO BY SUE SHEPHERD

Gluten-Free Cooking

The Gluten-Free Kitchen

THE COMPLETE
Low-FODMAP Diet

A Revolutionary Plan for Managing IBS and Other Digestive Disorders

SUE SHEPHERD, PhD, and **PETER GIBSON, MD**

Foreword by William D. Chey, MD
Food photography by Mark O'Meara

THE EXPERIMENT
NEW YORK

THE COMPLETE LOW-FODMAP DIET: *A Revolutionary Plan for Managing IBS and Other Digestive Disorders*

Text copyright © Sue Shepherd and Peter Gibson, 2011, 2013
Foreword © William D. Chey, 2013
Photographs copyright © Mark O'Meara, 2011

First published in somewhat different form by Penguin Group (Australia), 2011

Versions of the Brownies recipe (page 208) and Rhubarb and Raspberry Crumble recipe (page 243) previously appeared in *Low FODMAP Recipes* by Sue Shepherd (Penguin Group (Australia): Melbourne, 2013), and are reprinted with permission. A version of the Shepherd's Pie recipe (page 133) previously appeared in *The Gluten-Free Kitchen* by Sue Shepherd (Penguin Group (Australia): Melbourne, 2009), and is reprinted with permission.

All rights reserved. Except for brief passages quoted in newspaper, magazine, radio, television, or online reviews, no portion of this book may be reproduced, distributed, or transmitted in any form or by any means, electronic or mechanical, including photocopying, recording, or information storage or retrieval system, without the prior written permission of the publisher.

Many of the designations used by manufacturers and sellers to distinguish their products are claimed as trademarks. Where those designations appear in this book and The Experiment was aware of a trademark claim, the designations have been capitalized.

The Experiment, LLC
260 Fifth Avenue
New York, NY 10001-6408
www.theexperimentpublishing.com

This book contains the opinions and ideas of its authors. It is intended to provide helpful and informative material on the subjects addressed in the book. It is sold with the understanding that the authors and publisher are not engaged in rendering medical, health, or any other kind of personal professional services in the book. The authors and publisher specifically disclaim all responsibility for any liability, loss, or risk—personal or otherwise—that is incurred as a consequence, directly or indirectly, of the use and application of any of the contents of this book.

The Experiment's books are available at special discounts when purchased in bulk for premiums and sales promotions as well as for fundraising or educational use. For details, contact us at info@theexperimentpublishing.com.

Library of Congress Cataloging-in-Publication Data

Shepherd, Sue.
  The complete low-FODMAP diet : a revolutionary plan for managing IBS and other digestive disorders / Sue Shepherd and Peter Gibson ; food photography by Mark O'Meara.
     pages cm
  Includes bibliographical references and index.
  ISBN 978-1-61519-080-5 (pbk.) -- ISBN 978-1-61519-173-4 (ebook)
1. Irritable colon--Diet therapy--Recipes. 2. Intestines--Diseases--Diet therapy--Recipes. I. Gibson, P. R. II. Title. III. Title: Complete low-fermentable oligosaccharides, disaccharides, monosaccharides, and polyols diet.
  RC862.I77S48 2013
  616.3'440654--dc23
                                                    2013012045

ISBN 978-1-61519-080-5
Ebook ISBN 978-1-61519-173-4

Cover design by Susi Oberhelman
Cover photograph of vegetables © Skylines | Shutterstock
Text design by Pauline Neuwirth, Neuwirth & Associates, Inc.

Manufactured in the United States of America
Distributed by Workman Publishing Company, Inc.
Distributed simultaneously in Canada by Thomas Allen and Son Ltd.

First North American edition published August 2013
10 9 8 7 6 5 4 3 2 1

CONTENTS

CHAPTER SEVEN
Making the Low-FODMAP Diet Easier

CHAPTER EIGHT
Special Occasions and the Low-FODMAP Diet

PART TWO
Low-FODMAP Recipes

Appetizers and Light Meals

Salads

Soups, Stews, and Curries

Casseroles and Baked Dishes

Pasta, Noodles, and Rice

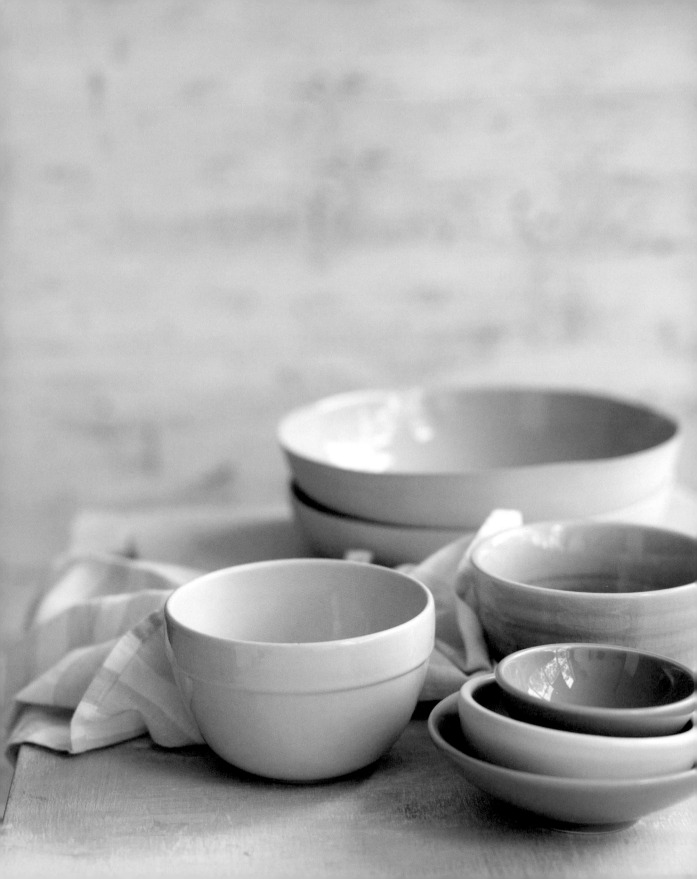

DURING MY MEDICAL training in gastro-enterology at the University of Michigan from 1990 to 1993, I learned about irritable bowel syndrome or IBS, a common condition defined by the presence of symptoms including abdominal pain or discomfort, bloating, and altered bowel habits. I was struck by research reporting that roughly one in ten people suffered from symptoms of IBS and that it was one of the most common causes of work absenteeism. As I gained experience caring for patients with IBS, the level of suffering they endured became more and more apparent.

Despite evidence that up to two thirds of IBS sufferers associated eating a meal with onset or aggravation of their IBS symptoms, the prevailing "wisdom" at that time was that food played little role in IBS. Rather, most doctors believed that IBS was caused by abnormal activity and sensitivity in the gastrointestinal (GI) tract, with significant contributions from psychological factors like depression and anxiety. At the time of my training, doctors received little to no formal training in the role of diet and nutrition in the management of gastrointestinal disorders such as IBS. We routinely told patients to eat smaller meals, reduce intake of fatty or greasy foods, and eat more fiber. These recommendations were the standard of care for IBS sufferers well into the new century. Unfortunately, both patients and physicians have grown increasingly frustrated with the inconsistent results yielded by these recommendations. Despite this, little has

changed in regards to physicians' training in nutrition and diet. The difficulties in obtaining helpful dietary advice from physicians and other medical providers and the growing interest in more holistic approaches to the management of IBS have led many patients to take matters into their own hands, self-imposing highly restrictive and potentially dangerous diets. A number of "exclusion" diets for IBS have received attention over the years but very few have been based upon a clear scientific rationale or found to be effective in high-quality clinical research studies.

The low-FODMAP diet has managed to break this mold and, in so doing, is gradually changing the way that patients and physicians view the role of diet in the management of IBS. I remember first reading about fermentable oligosaccharides, disaccharides, monosaccharides, and polyols, or FODMAPs, in a research paper published by Sue Shepherd and Peter Gibson in 2005. I was intrigued by the FODMAP concept because it made scientific and practical sense. I am quite proud to say that the University of Michigan was one of the first major US medical centers to adopt the low-FODMAP diet as a routine part of treating our patients with IBS. Initial discussions with our physicians and dieticians were typically met with palpable skepticism ("it's way too restrictive," "it's too complicated," "patients will never do it," "just another fad diet," "I don't believe it will work"). However, as patients returned with story after story of remarkable improvement, this skepticism was quickly replaced by enthusiasm and praise. Concurrent with the gradual adoption of the low-FODMAP approach has been a dramatic shift in the behavior of our providers from viewing the low-FODMAP diet as a "rescue" strategy intended only for those that had failed all other therapies to now viewing the diet as an *evidence-based*, *first-line* treatment strategy.

I have no doubt that patients and medical providers will benefit from the easy-to-understand, practical information provided in *The Complete Low-FODMAP Diet*. The availability of this useful resource will help affected patients and interested medical providers to better understand and incorporate the low-FODMAP diet into their lives in a safe, medically responsible, and tasty way.

Bon appétit!

WILLIAM D. CHEY, MD, AGAF, FACG, FACP, RFF, is Professor of Medicine, Director of the GI Physiology Laboratory, and Co-Director of the Michigan Bowel Control Program at the University of Michigan. He also runs a clinical research group, serves as Co-editor-in-Chief of the American Journal of Gastroenterology, and and is on the Board of Trustees of the American College of Gastroenterology and the Board of Directors of the Rome Foundation and Advisory Board of the International Foundation for Functional Gastrointestinal Disorders (IFFGD).

ACROSS THE WORLD, one in ten people suffer from irritable bowel syndrome (IBS)—a chronic condition whose symptoms include abdominal pain and bloating, excessive gas, and diarrhea or constipation or both, often on a daily basis. While doctors are good at diagnosing it, they don't have much of a track record in fixing the problem.

If you have IBS or suffer from one or more food intolerances or other persistent digestive trouble and are sick of feeling unwell, then this is the book for you. The low-FODMAP diet is the first program scientifically proven to relieve the symptoms of IBS, and it can also help with other digestive conditions, including Crohn's disease, ulcerative colitis, and celiac disease (alongside a fully gluten-free diet) The program has transformed the lives of many people and could work for you, too.

FODMAP is the collective abbreviation for a group of fermentable, poorly absorbed short-chain carbohydrates that provide fast food for bowel bacteria and may cause digestive discomfort. **FODMAP** stands for **F**ermentable **O**ligosaccharides, **D**isaccharides, **M**onosaccharides, **A**nd **P**olyols.

If this seems too wordy to get your head around, remember that *saccharide* is simply another word for sugar. Oligosaccharides, disaccharides, and monosaccharides are carbohydrates made up of sugar molecules, and polyols are what we call sugar alcohols, sugar molecules with an alcohol side-chain.

We will describe FODMAPs and the low-FODMAP diet in greater detail later in this book. We'll tell you which foods are safe, which foods you can eat in moderation, and which foods you may need to restrict completely—and we'll help you adjust to a personalized low-FODMAP diet that accommodates your individual food intolerances and preferences. For now, here are some key points about the diet:

- It has been scientifically proven.
- It provides all the nutrients you need.
- It can help you stay symptom-free in the long term—some people have lived symptom-free on their individualized diet for months and even years.
- It won't cure your IBS, but it will help to prevent triggering your symptoms.

If you have been troubled by IBS in the past, we feel confident that you will find great relief in following the low-FODMAP diet outlined in this book. Once you're up and running, you might need to keep referring to the book as you go, but with time the diet will become second nature to you. Soon you'll simply feel better than you ever did, without having to put too much effort into the "how." And using the recipes in this book will help make your process of adaptation to the diet much smoother.

Sincere best wishes for good health.

Dr. Sue Shepherd and Dr. Peter Gibson

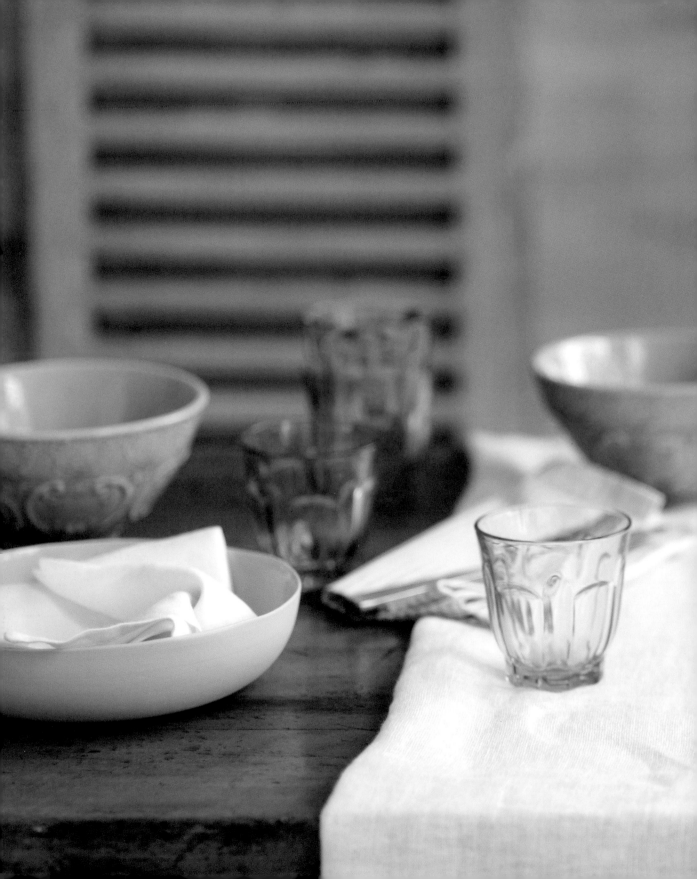

PART ONE

All About the Low-FODMAP Diet

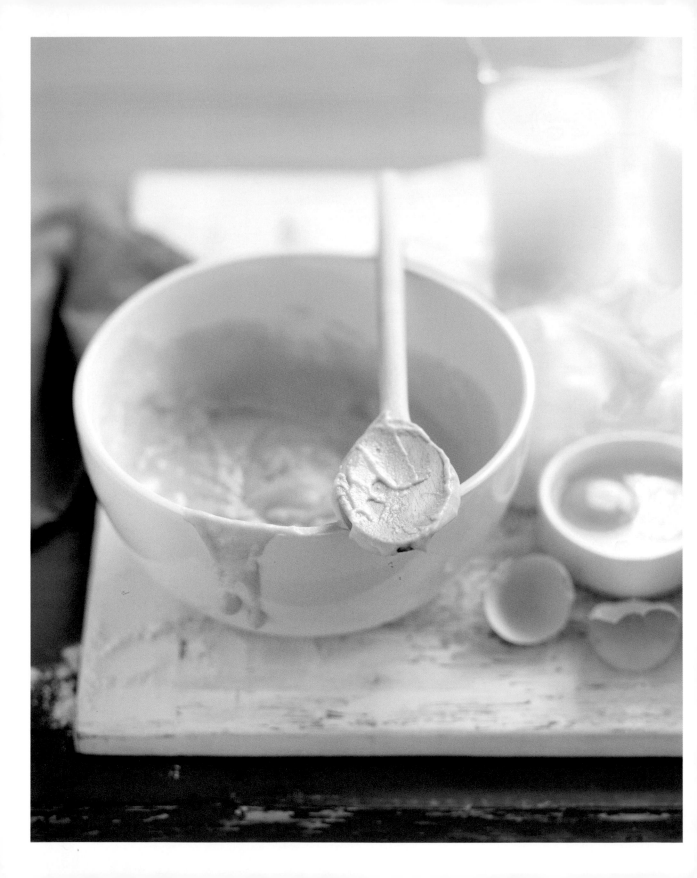

How Food Can Trigger Gut Symptoms

CHAPTER ONE

THE HUMAN GUT

In order to understand the various disorders and symptoms related to the foods we eat, it is helpful first to understand the gut, its structure (anatomy), and how it works. The gut is also known as the gastrointestinal tract, the digestive tract, or the alimentary tract. The main job of the gut is to take in food, break it down so that energy and nutrients can be extracted, and then expel the remaining waste. In the process, the gut also has to protect the body from exposure to things that are toxic or not good for it in other ways.

It is easiest to think of the gut as a hollow tube that runs from the mouth to the anus. This long tube, which averages about twenty feet, is made up of many layers and divided into various parts, each of which performs a specialized function. After you swallow your food, it enters the *esophagus,* which pushes the food down into your *stomach,* where food is liquefied and sterilized, and digestion begins. The semidigested food then passes into the *small intestine* or *small bowel*, where food is broken down into its simple building blocks (sugars, amino acids, and fatty acids) and the nutrients are absorbed. The small intestine has three sections with different roles in breaking down food and absorbing nutrients: the *duodenum*, the *ileum*, and the *jejunum*.

The leftovers then move into the *large intestine* or *large bowel,* where salts and water are reabsorbed as the contents pass slowly

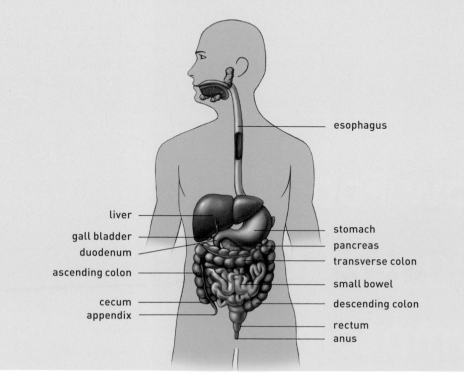

esophagus

liver
gall bladder
duodenum
ascending colon

cecum
appendix

stomach
pancreas
transverse colon

small bowel

descending colon

rectum
anus

around the several components of the large bowel: the *cecum*, the *ascending colon*, the *transverse colon*, the *descending colon*, and the *rectum*. The contents are packaged into stools that are then excreted via the *anus*.

While some *intestinal bacteria* are present in the small bowel, the large bowel contains vast numbers of them. These bacteria feast on undigested or indigestible food, producing short-chain fatty acids that nourish the lining of the large bowel and gas that contributes to flatulence.

The whole process of mixing and moving contents around the gut is controlled by a complex of nerves in the wall of the gut known as the *enteric nervous system* (ENS) or "gut brain." The ENS senses what is going into the gut and controls its motility (i.e., muscle activity and its coordination). Although the ENS is connected to and can be influenced by the brain (and vice versa), it can function without these connections, using its own networks of neurons (nerves). The brain can influence both our perception of what is happening in the gut and also the activity, or "tuning," of the ENS. The interaction between the brain and gut is different for each individual and can depend on factors such as state of mind, surrounding environment, the presence or absence of distractions, and past experiences, as well as the gut's sensitivity to stimuli. For more on the human gut and the ENS, see the comprehensive information on this book's website, www.thelowfodmapdiet.com.

This book focuses on a diet-based management plan for irritable bowel syndrome and other digestive conditions. But before we get to that, we would like to describe some important information about digestion and conditions that can cause digestive symptoms.

Gut reactions to food

As you can see, digestion is a complex process that involves many parts working in harmony. When one or more parts of the gut is "out of tune," negative reactions may result. The terms *food allergy*, *food hypersensitivity*, and *food intolerance* are often used interchangeably and quite incorrectly. There are two very different types of adverse reaction to food:

1. *Immunological reactions.* These are reactions to a protein in the food and involve the immune system. This type of reaction, often called a *food allergy* or *food hypersensitivity*, is quite uncommon (affecting about one in fifty people). These reactions are always reproducible, reliable responses to particular foods that occur even after consuming only a small amount of the food.

2. *Non-immunological reactions.* These reactions do not involve the immune system and are usually referred to as *food intolerances*. They are very common (affecting about one in five people). These reactions can vary and depend on the amount consumed, timing of the meal, and other meals consumed in that day.

CELIAC DISEASE

WHAT IS IT?

Celiac disease is an extreme example of food hypersensitivity. It is the result of an immune reaction to gluten that severely injures the body, and has been called an autoimmune disease (because the body turns on itself). Gluten is the main protein in wheat, rye, and barley. Some people with celiac also react to avenin, the protein in oats. When people with celiac disease eat foods containing gluten, the lining of their bowel is damaged by the white blood cells of their immune system (not by antibodies as in a food allergy).

SYMPTOMS

These range from none at all to nausea, flatulence, bloating, altered bowel habits (constipation or diarrhea or a combination of both), fatigue of varying severity, and even skin rashes and liver or neurological problems. It can cause vitamin and mineral deficiencies (particularly of iron, folic acid, zinc, and vitamin D) and can also cause malnutrition through weight loss and loss of muscle mass (although this is less common these days).

DIAGNOSIS

The diagnosis of celiac disease is through blood tests to measure certain types of antibodies that occur only in people with celiac disease. If blood tests are positive, then an upper GI endoscopy (an examination of the upper gut using an endoscope) is performed and tissue samples are taken from the duodenum (the beginning of the small bowel). The samples are examined to see if the bowel lining is damaged in the pattern typical of celiac disease.

Before the tests, patients are asked to consume foods that contain gluten (e.g., the equivalent of four slices of bread per day) for at least six weeks. If the tests are negative (normal) but you have been following a gluten-free diet, neither you nor your doctor will be any the wiser about whether you have celiac disease, and you will need to undergo the tests again. It is *essential* to have these tests before you start a gluten-free diet.

TREATMENT

The only way to treat celiac disease is with a gluten-free diet for life: no wheat, rye, barley, and products derived from them, ever. Some people react to oats and need to restrict these, too. Oats tend to be contaminated with gluten-containing grains, so even those who need not avoid oats entirely should consume only certified gluten-free oats. Eating gluten-free usually requires a major change in diet, but as a rule, the gut symptoms, fatigue, and other problems disappear over time and the bowel slowly heals. Many complications can occur if celiac disease is not recognized and treated, including thinning of the bones (osteoporosis), infertility, miscarriage, liver disease, and even lymphoma, a cancer of the lymph nodes. This is why it is so important to investigate the cause of gut symptoms.

About one in twenty people diagnosed with irritable bowel syndrome has celiac disease. A gluten-free diet is usually a very effective treatment for IBS symptoms for those who have celiac disease.

If you are diagnosed with celiac disease and suffer from gut symptoms despite following a strict gluten-free diet, talk to a registered dietitian about whether the low-FODMAP diet would help you.

FOOD HYPERSENSITIVITIES

Food hypersensitivities, including food allergies, are immune reactions to a specific component in a food (called an allergen), which is almost always a protein. Symptoms include hives, asthma, a runny nose, and mouth-swelling. The foods that most commonly cause adverse reactions are shellfish, eggs, fish, milk, tree nuts and peanuts, sesame seeds, soy, wheat, rye, barley, and oats. With food allergies, the body reacts to the allergen by producing an antibody to it or with other immune responses. The symptoms experienced depend on the immunological reaction within the body.

Food allergies

In a true food allergy, the body makes antibodies known as immunoglobulin E (IgE). When the antibodies and the allergen meet, it triggers the release of histamine and other defensive chemicals into the body. These chemicals can cause reactions in the mouth, gut, skin, lungs, heart, and blood vessels. Symptoms can include itching, burning and swelling of the mouth, runny nose, skin rash, diarrhea and abdominal cramps, breathing difficulties, vomiting, and nausea. In severe cases they can be life threatening—a reaction called *anaphylaxis*, in which the circulatory system collapses. People with food allergies may experience gut symptoms, but they are usually minor compared with their other symptoms.

Non-allergic food hypersensitivities

Immune responses that do not involve IgE antibodies are often referred to as *food hypersensitivities*. The symptoms related to food hypersensitivity may only affect the gut. These reactions are not easy to diagnose, because they don't usually produce antibodies that can be detected in a blood test. One way to help determine whether certain food proteins are causing specific immune responses is to inject them under the skin and look for reactions. But unfortunately these tests don't tell us what is causing the gut symptoms, because the response to proteins in the gut is often very different from that under the skin. The current method of detecting food hypersensitivities is placing the patients on a bland elimination diet, and then, if their symptoms improve, "challenging" with specific food components to see which cause renewed symptoms. This can be a very long process.

This book and the low-FODMAP diet are not designed to treat food allergies or hypersensitivities. If you think you might have a food allergy or intolerance, contact the allergy centers of major hospitals, the National Institute of Allergy and Infectious Diseases (NIAID), or Food Allergy Research & Education (FARE).

FOOD INTOLERANCES

Unlike food allergy and hypersensitivity, *food intolerance* does not involve the immune system. Food intolerances are the most common trigger of gut symptoms, but they can also cause other symptoms, such as headaches and fatigue. This book and the low-FODMAP diet are designed to help sufferers of food intolerances. There are two main ways that food intolerances can manifest themselves in gut symptoms:

1. By inducing bowel distension, and thus triggering gut symptoms. This is by far the most common way in which symptoms occur, and the FODMAP sugars (see Chapter 3) are common triggers.

2. By responding to foods containing high levels of bioactive substances and food chemicals that either occur naturally in foods or are added during food processing. Common examples include caffeine, salicylates, amines, glutamate, and colorings and preservatives. Please see the American Academy of Allergy, Asthma and Immunology website (www.aaaai.org) for further information.

IRRITABLE BOWEL SYNDROME

Irritable bowel syndrome (IBS) is one of a group of conditions called *functional gastrointestinal disorders*, which are the most common gut conditions, together affecting about one in five people. *Functional* means that they cause disturbances in the *function* of the gut but don't have any identifiable physical features,

such as ulcers, inflammation, thickening of tissues, lumps and bumps, or abnormal blood tests, all of which would indicate a different condition. The diagnosis of functional disorders, including IBS, relies upon the types of symptoms experienced and their context, such as how long they have been experienced and when they occur.

Most people with food allergies do not have IBS. Food hypersensitivity can be an underlying problem in some people who have IBS, but the symptoms of IBS are most commonly triggered by a food intolerance. If you suffer from IBS, you very likely have a food intolerance—so this book is for you.

The symptoms of IBS

Sufferers of IBS can experience a broad range of symptoms, including abdominal pain and discomfort, bloating, changes in bowel habits, heartburn, nausea, overfullness, and so on. Some of these symptoms originate in the upper gut (the esophagus and stomach) while others originate in the bowel. Other symptoms or perceived symptoms can include excessive gas, unsatisfied defecation (incomplete emptying), passage of slimy mucus into the toilet bowl, a noisy abdomen (the noises are called *borborygmi*), and pain in the rectum. Tiredness is also common and its severity usually depends on that of the bowel symptoms. Muscle aches and pains (called *fibromyalgia*) occur in some people, while others experience an "irritable bladder" (urinary frequency and urgency).

Definition and diagnosis of IBS

The official medical definition of IBS is part of what is called the "Rome III" classification. It says that people can be diagnosed with IBS if they have suffered symptoms of a functional gut disorder for at least six months, and have experienced for at least three months of the year mid- or lower abdominal pain or discomfort associated with abdominal bloating or distension, along with changes in bowel habits (diarrhea, constipation, or both). The sufferer need not have experienced all these symptoms and they need not have occurred together, but they often do. The time requirements are used to differentiate IBS from acute, isolated stomach trouble that everyone has from time to time.

A typical diagnostic process is as follows:

1. *Identification of symptoms suggestive of IBS.* Your doctor will look for the "ABC" of IBS—**a**bdominal pain or discomfort, **b**loating, and **c**hanges in bowel habits.

2. *Identification of other symptoms.* Your doctor will try to identify "alarm symptoms" or red flags that may indicate another condition rather than IBS. For example, if the symptoms started after age fifty, or if there is blood in the stools, fever, weight loss of more than ten pounds (five kilograms), symptoms that wake you up at night, or a strong family history of colorectal cancer, then your doctor will investigate the possibility of inflammatory colorectal disease, cancer, or other causes, depending upon the situation.

3. *Examination for signs of illness.* IBS is seldom associated with any physical indications of illness.

4. *Provisional diagnosis of IBS.*

INFLAMMATORY BOWEL DISEASE (IBD)

Some people who suffer from IBS-like symptoms are diagnosed with inflammatory bowel disease (IBD). Unlike IBS and other functional gut disorders, IBD is an illness in which the bowel becomes chronically inflamed. This may cause diarrhea that can be bloody, abdominal pain, tiredness, and many other symptoms. There are two main types of IBD: Crohn's disease (which can affect any part of the gut) and ulcerative colitis (which affects only the large bowel).

The causes for these conditions are not known, and treatment is directed toward controlling the inflammation and preventing it from returning. Dietary change typically plays only a very small role in this aspect of treatment. Those with IBD whose bowel inflammation is well controlled but whose symptoms continue may also find the low-FODMAP diet a useful tool. See page 58 for more on incorporating the diet into your overall treatment plan.

5. *Further investigation.* This should always include a blood test for celiac disease and, in some people, extra blood tests with or without an endoscopic examination of the stomach and duodenum (called an *endoscopy*)

and of the colon (called a *colonoscopy*). The necessity of extra tests depends upon your age, the pattern of symptoms, and the presence of alarm symptoms as above.

6. *Definitive diagnosis of IBS.* If the tests reveal no other potential cause for the symptoms, then you will be diagnosed with IBS.

Once the diagnosis is complete, you and your doctor will start working on treatment for your IBS. One of the best ways we know of for treating the symptoms of IBS is following the low-FODMAP diet, which has been proven to relieve symptoms in three quarters of IBS sufferers. For more about the low-FODMAP diet and how to incorporate it into your life, see Chapter 3 (page 24) and Chapter 4 (page 38).

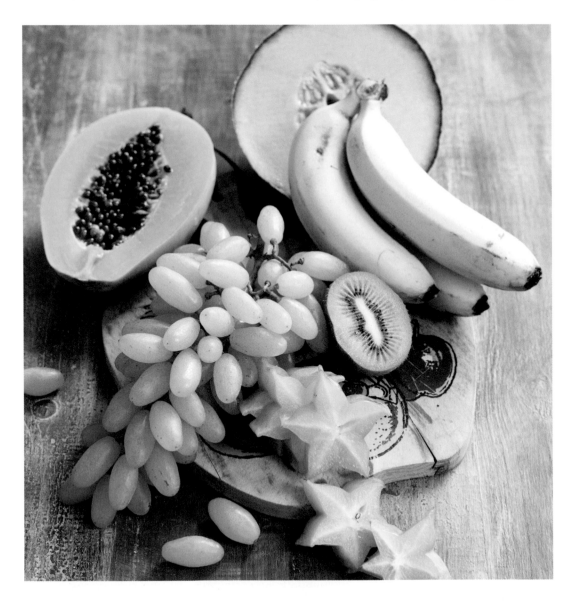

What Is IBS?

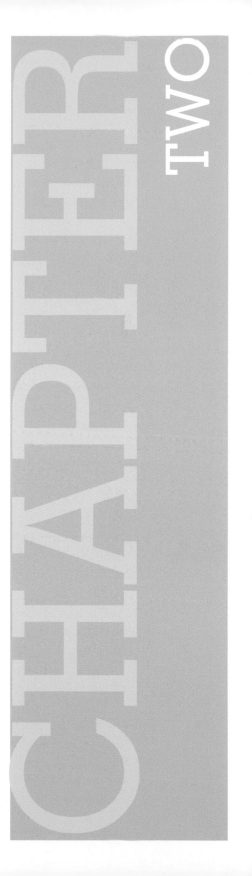

CHAPTER TWO

What causes IBS?

We really don't know why some people get IBS and others do not, but one day a single cause might be recognized and a cure found. As far as we can tell, there is no simple infection or other cause that brings about IBS. What we *do* know is that the "tuning" of the complex nervous system that controls the gut, called the *enteric nervous system* (ENS), is involved. When the ENS is badly tuned, the result can be an extrasensitive nerve response in the gut (called *visceral hypersensitivity*) and/or abnormalities in how the gut moves and deals with its contents. But what actually puts the ENS out of tune and what keeps it out of tune is largely a mystery.

It seems that many factors can contribute to the development of IBS, including:

1. *Genetic factors.* We know from studies of twins that genes play at least some role in IBS, and it is not unusual for IBS to occur within a family.

2. *Gut infections*. For example, when large communities have been infected by a waterborne germ that causes severe diarrhea, many people have later developed IBS (with diarrhea as the main symptom). This is called *postinfectious IBS*, and people who suffer from it may have an ongoing very mild inflammation of the gut. Unfortunately, anti-inflammatory drugs seem to have no benefit.

3. *Stress and other psychological factors.* These can affect the ENS by altering how the nerve signals from the gut are transmitted to and interpreted by the brain and spinal cord. The links between the brain and the ENS are collectively called the *brain–gut axis*. Disturbances in this axis can contribute to IBS and can also affect anyone.

4. *Abnormal balance of gut bacteria.* Disturbances in the balance of the bacteria that live in the large bowel may contribute to IBS. This is called *dysbiosis*, and there are different theories about how it might affect the bowel or why it occurs:
   ➤ *Small intestinal bacterial overgrowth (SIBO)*—One new and quite controversial theory is that IBS is caused by the growth of too many bacteria in the small bowel.
   ➤ *Food-related causes*—What we eat influences the relative number of different types of bacteria in our bowel. Whether these changes can actually cause IBS symptoms by changing the way the ENS is tuned is the subject of ongoing research.
   ➤ *Early childhood exposure*—We develop our own set of bacterial types in our bowel at an early age, and it is possible that in some people an interaction between these bacteria and exposure to aspects of the environment (not just food) dictates how their ENS is tuned.

5. *Joint hypermobility.* About one in five people has *joint hypermobility syndrome*. This refers to having joints with greater flexibility, such as being double-jointed or able not only to touch your toes but also to put the palms of your hands on the ground.

It has recently been found that this condition is associated with a higher chance of having IBS. It is assumed to be related to the relative laxness of the tissues in the gut—they tend to distend more (see "Bloating and distension," below).

What causes the symptoms of IBS?

Here are a few facts about the origin of the most common symptoms of IBS: bloating and distension, abdominal pain and discomfort, changes in bowel habits, variations in the characteristics of stools, excessive flatulence, a noisy abdomen, and fatigue.

BLOATING AND DISTENSION

Bloating is defined as the *feeling* of increased pressure in the abdomen, whereas distension is a *measurable change* in the circumference of the abdomen. Bloating and distension typically increase for IBS sufferers during the day and after eating. Distension and bloating can be experienced simultaneously or separately. By far the majority of bloating appears to originate in the bowel. How much distension occurs also depends upon unconscious reflexes that occur when the bowel distends (see page 15).

There are only three things that can distend the bowel: solids, liquids, and gases. Excesses of these in the bowel cause bloating and distension because they increase the size of the bowel, causing it to take up much more space within the abdomen.

Solids

The only place where any solid matter is retained is the large bowel. Excessive amounts of solids, as may occur in constipation, can cause distension. The large bowel is built to accommodate a fairly large capacity, so it handles distension better than the small bowel. The best way to determine whether the large bowel is overfull is by X-raying the abdomen. And the best way to determine whether this is contributing to the feeling of bloating is to clear the bowel out (under medical supervision) and see if this relieves the bloating.

Liquids and gases

Excessive amounts of liquid and gas in the bowel, particularly the last three feet of the small bowel and the first parts of the large bowel, are the most common cause of distension, particularly when the distension and bloating vary in severity during the day. How much liquid is retained in the bowel and how much gas is produced depend largely on what food is eaten.

During the digestion process, water and salts are drawn into the body through the walls of the small and large bowel (a process called *absorption*). If this process is disturbed by illnesses such as a gut infection, pancreatic disease, celiac disease, or inflammatory bowel disease, more liquid will remain in the bowel, which is why diarrhea is often caused by these conditions.

One way the body maintains its balance is by ensuring that the total number of molecules in bodily fluids per unit volume (e.g., per milliliter) remains constant. If you ingest a lot of molecules that cannot be absorbed from the bowel into the bloodstream, the only way your body can keep the number of molecules per unit volume the same is to increase the amount of water retained in your bowel. The bowel usually responds to all this extra fluid by increasing the speed at which it propels the contents, which may lead to diarrhea. Our diet typically includes many foods containing sugars that are poorly absorbed in the small bowel. All these sugars in the bowel result in more water being retained there. We have called such sugars FODMAPs (see page 24), and our diet for IBS sufferers is based on avoidance of these sugars.

Gas is produced by intestinal bacteria as they feed on unabsorbed food molecules that reach the large bowel. The process by which they do this is called *fermentation*, and many of us know from making bread or beer that fermentation generates lots of gas. When bacteria ferment carbohydrates (such as sugars), the gases produced are mostly hydrogen and carbon dioxide, although many also produce methane. These odorless gases are produced in large amounts. A small amount of carbon dioxide will travel down the remaining part of the gut and be expelled as flatulence, but most of the carbon dioxide produced is either used by bacteria for other purposes or absorbed into the bloodstream across the lining of the large bowel, taken up to the lungs, and exhaled. Likewise, some of the hydrogen is incorporated by the bacteria into short-chain fatty acids, converted (with carbon dioxide) into methane, or used to make hydrogen sulfide. The rest will be absorbed into the bloodstream and exhaled through the lungs.

FODMAPs

Many carbohydrates in food are poorly digested and are not absorbed by the small bowel. Dietary fiber is one example. Some fiber, known as *insoluble fiber*, cannot be fermented by bacteria, while other fiber, known as *soluble fiber*, can be fermented by bacteria. Some simple sugars, oligosaccharides (short chains of sugars), and sugar alcohols are also indigestible and/or cannot be absorbed by the bowel, but can be broken down by intestinal bacteria to produce gas.

One way to reduce the amount of gas in the bowel is to eat a minimal amount of carbohydrates, except for those that are readily digested, such as sucrose (cane sugar) or glucose—although we do not recommend eating too much of these, as doing so can lead to weight gain, cavities, and other health problems. A much better and more practical approach is to determine which carbohydrates are the major contributors to the production of gas in the bowel and to restrict them. These are the carbohydrates that are easily and rapidly fermented by bacteria (they could be considered bacterial "fast food")—the molecules we call FODMAPs. We know from our studies that FODMAPs can cause diarrhea, gas production, and excess flatulence. We have also found that the low-FODMAP diet reduces bloating, distension, and flatulence in at least three out of every four people with IBS.

ABDOMINAL PAIN AND DISCOMFORT

The major cause of abdominal pain and discomfort in IBS is distension of the bowel. How

WHY DON'T WE ALL SUFFER FROM IBS?

We all eat FODMAPs and produce gas, so why do only some people get IBS? There are five possible reasons:

1. *How much gas we make.* This depends upon the types of bacteria living in our bowel and how they dispose of the gas. Everyone's bowel has a different combination of bacteria, and some bacteria are vigorous fermenters, while others produce less gas.

2. *The visceral sensitivity of our bowel.* This is more pronounced in some people. The sensation of bloating depends upon how our ENS is tuned (see page 5) and what degree of distension occurs before we experience discomfort.

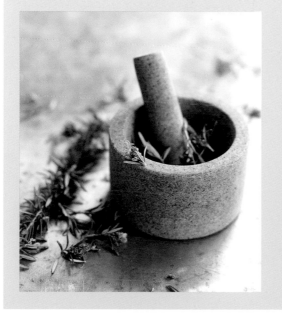

3. *How well our abdominal wall can move gas once it is formed.* Usually, when a lot of gas is introduced into the bowel, this stimulates the digestive tract to move the gas rapidly down the bowel until it is expelled as flatulence. In some people with IBS, however, the gas just sits around in the bowel, causing more distension.

4. *How well our bowel reacts to distension.* Typically, when the bowel is distended, our stomach muscles tighten automatically, without any input from the brain, so that our abdomen does not stick out. In some people with IBS, however, these reflex responses are very weak. When the bowel is distended, the diaphragm (a large muscle that sits below the lungs) usually becomes more relaxed, allowing more space for the bowel in the abdomen. For people with IBS, however, bowel distension may lead to contraction and, therefore, flattening of the diaphragm, which causes more obvious distension and greater discomfort.

5. *Our awareness of signals from the gut and how we interpret them.* We interpret signals from the gut differently under different circumstances. Our perceptions do change according to our levels of stress and anxiety and according to what is going on in our lives. This is also part of the brain–gut axis in action.

much pain and discomfort is experienced depends on the sensitivity of the nerve endings in the bowel. If they are very sensitive, we say the person has *visceral hypersensitivity*.

We can determine whether someone has visceral hypersensitivity by doing what we call *barostat studies*. One study involves inserting a tube with an attached inflatable balloon into the rectum via the anus. In people without IBS, we can inflate the balloon quite a bit before they experience pain or discomfort, but most people with IBS will experience pain with much less inflation of the balloon. These experiments show that people with IBS require less distension before their nerves send messages to their brain to indicate that they are in pain. In other words, people with IBS appear to have more sensitive nerve endings that react earlier to small amounts of stimulation, so that they experience pain when someone without IBS would not. Another cause of abdominal discomfort is severe contraction of the muscles in the gut wall, causing cramping abdominal pain.

The important feature of bowel pain is that we feel it over a large area of the lower, middle, or upper abdomen, but can seldom say exactly where it's coming from. Unlike the skin, where there are lots of pain receptors so that our conscious brain knows exactly where the source of pain is, the abdomen has only general pain receptors, which means that our conscious brain can only recognize that something is happening inside a large part of the abdomen. Usually (but not always), pain from the stomach and duodenum is felt in the upper abdomen, from the small bowel in the middle abdomen and from the large bowel in the lower abdomen.

CHANGES IN BOWEL HABITS

The nature of our bowel actions—loose as in diarrhea or hard and dry as in constipation—depends largely on their water content.

Diarrhea means that the amount of liquid in the bowel has exceeded the ability of the bowel to dry out its contents. There can be three main reasons for this:

1. The amount of liquid coming from the small bowel is too great.
2. The drying-out mechanism is impaired (e.g., when the colon is inflamed).
3. The speed at which the contents are traveling through the bowel is too fast for drying out to occur (the ENS is driving the muscles too vigorously).

Likewise, constipation can be due to:

1. Too little liquid entering the bowel.
2. Too much drying out, because the contents of the bowel are moving too slowly or bowel emptying is too poorly coordinated.
3. Not emptying the bowel as soon as the urge occurs.

The amount of water we drink has some influence here: If we do not drink enough, we absorb more salts and water from the bowel, and the chance of constipation increases. But we cannot readily increase the amount of water in the large bowel simply by drinking more water, since this water will be absorbed higher up and the excess will be passed in the urine. In other words, if you are constipated, you should make sure you do not get dehydrated, but drinking several liters of water per day will not give any additional benefit.

Transit time

The time it takes for the bowel contents to move from the beginning to the end of the large bowel is called the *transit time*. One factor affecting transit time is the inherent way the ENS is tuned. In some people, transit time will be long, and their normal bowel pattern will be, for example, five times a week with fairly firm stools. Others have a shorter transit time, normally going two to three times a day and producing softer stools.

From this baseline, other factors can change the transit time. One is the nature of the diet. If it contains little fiber, things will move sluggishly along the bowel and constipation might result. In such situations, a switch to a high-fiber diet or taking fiber supplements would work very well. If, on the other hand, the diet contains a large amount of poorly absorbed sugars (FODMAPs), the ENS may respond by directing the colon muscles to expel the bowel contents and the transit time will then become very short.

It is worth noting that opiate drugs (also known as narcotics) such as codeine can be particularly constipating because they slow the bowel down and so increase the transit time. So if you experience abdominal pain due to IBS, opiate drugs are not a good option.

VARIATIONS IN THE CHARACTERISTICS OF STOOLS

People with IBS often question the features of their stools. These can include:

- **Color**—The color of the stools does vary, but these variations are not usually significant in IBS.
- **Shape**—Ribbon-like or stringy stools, usually associated with straining, indicate constipation. Pellets like rabbit droppings also indicate constipation. Floating stools can indicate a good fiber intake.
- **Bits and pieces within the stool**—Sometimes people notice tomato skins, corn kernels, or seeds in their stools and think this indicates a problem with their digestion, but this is usually only because they have never looked closely before. Many people's stools look like this.
- **Mucus**—It is normal to pass mucus, the slimy stuff that coats the bowel wall, with your stools, and it usually has no serious implications.
- **Blood**—Any blood in the stool warrants a visit to the doctor. It is not part of IBS.

EXCESSIVE FLATULENCE

Farting is normal: Healthy women fart on average seven times a day, and healthy men fourteen times a day. We can expel as much as two liters of gas a day; up to half of that might be swallowed air, but the rest is produced in the colon through bacterial fermentation.

There are generally two complaints made about farts:

1. **Frequency.** The way to reduce the volume of gas expelled is to reduce the supply of carbohydrates to the bacteria by avoiding gas-producing foods rich in FODMAPs, soluble fiber,

- *Avoid excessive intake of fats, caffeine, and alcohol.* A low to moderate intake of the following is best both for long-term health and for minimizing the symptoms of IBS.
  - *Fat*—People with IBS have a lower threshold for bloating, discomfort, and pain after high-fat meals, so avoid rich, greasy food. Choose reduced-fat options when possible or only a small serving of a fatty food.
  - *Caffeine*—Caffeine is a stimulant and in susceptible people can make the digestive tract work faster, so contents move through more rapidly, sometimes leading to loose stools or diarrhea. It is best to limit caffeine-based beverages to, for example, no more than three cups of medium-strength coffee per day, and to spread intake out over the day.
  - *Alcohol*—Alcohol can worsen symptoms of IBS. Limit intake to moderate amounts in line with the USDA *Dietary Guidelines for Americans*, which recommends no more than one standard drink for females and two standard drinks for males per day. Try to have alcohol with food rather than on an empty stomach.
- *Avoid stress-filled meals.* Don't use mealtimes as a forum for difficult family discussions or work e-mails. Take time out to consciously enjoy your meal.
- *Don't skip meals—eat regularly.* People often skip meals as a way to avoid excessive calorie intake, but hunger might encourage rapid overeating at the next meal. Breakfast, in particular, is a meal that people are often tempted to skip, but eating breakfast is important. It

enables rehydration after many hours of no fluid intake and promotes a healthier intake of nutrients.

DRUGS

Medications generally have limited effectiveness in treating IBS overall, and as of this book's publication, no approved drug has been shown to relieve all IBS symptoms. Drugs can, however, play a definite role in treating specific troublesome symptoms of IBS. Your doctor may recommend medications in response to the major symptom that causes you distress, such as the following:

- *Abdominal cramping pains*—drugs that relieve spasms, such as mebeverine, anticholinergic drugs, or peppermint oil, would be the first choice, followed by antidepressant drugs, usually at low doses
- *Diarrhea*—drugs that slow the bowel, such as loperamide or diphenoxylate
- *Constipation*—a fiber supplement such as sterculia, or the use of laxatives such as Epsom salts or polyethylene glycol preparations
- *Sleep disturbance*—perhaps a tricyclic antidepressant
- *Anxiety and stress*—any of the antidepressants

Antibiotics have recently been shown to help some people with IBS where diarrhea is the predominant bowel habit. They are also sometimes used to treat small intestinal bacterial overgrowth, and do help in some cases, but the concept of bacterial overgrowth is very controversial. It is generally not a good idea to take antibiotics over a long period of time.

PSYCHOLOGICAL THERAPIES

Many people with IBS try psychological approaches like yoga and hypnotherapy (clinical hypnosis) to deal with issues such as anxiety and stress that may be contributing to their IBS. There is also now a body of evidence that these techniques help symptoms of IBS and work just as well or even better for people who are not so stressed. Cognitive behavior therapy with a trained psychologist or hypnotherapy with a trained hypnotherapist are less accessible, but there is very good evidence that they provide considerable benefit. "Gut-directed" hypnotherapy has been shown to have lasting benefits for people with IBS. How and why it works is not well understood, but it deserves attention. There is some evidence that it may reduce visceral hypersensitivity. If you're considering hypnotherapy, check the credentials and training of the hypnotherapist.

OTHER THERAPIES

Some people with IBS claim that these therapies have helped relieve their symptoms:

- **Probiotics**—These are friendly bacteria with supposed health benefits, usually various strains of *Lactobacillus* or *Bifidobacteria*, used alone or in combination. Many other types of bacteria (and even yeast) have also been marketed as probiotics. These have to be taken every day, as the bacteria do not remain in the gut for long. One good thing about probiotics is that they are unlikely to do any harm (apart from lightening the wallet—like many alternative therapies, they're not cheap and do not tend to be covered by insurance). Some do show evidence of benefit in well-designed studies, but often the benefit is small at best. If you want to try a probiotic preparation, find one that has clinical trial evidence of benefit (you can check this online). If you find it has benefits for you over, say, a four-week period, that is good and it can be continued. If you see no benefit when taking only a probiotic for your IBS, do not keep taking it.

- **Prebiotics**—These are carbohydrates, such as inulin (not to be confused with insulin) and fructose-oligosaccharide (also known as FOS or oligofructose), that, at low doses only, specifically encourage the growth of "good" bacteria and reduce the number of supposedly "bad" bacteria. There is no evidence that these help in IBS, and in fact, since they behave like or are FODMAPs, they are likely to cause *more* IBS symptoms. We currently do not recommend them.

- **Exercise**—Walking or doing simple exercises at the gym (rather than running marathons) may be beneficial.

- **Acupuncture**—Some people claim that acupuncture relieves their IBS symptoms, particularly abdominal pain. It remains unproven scientifically, but it is unlikely to do you any harm. If you're considering acupuncture, check the credentials and training of the acupuncturist.

- **Traditional Chinese medicine**—Although at least one study, out of Australia, has shown this to be effective for IBS, other studies have demonstrated little success, and there are so many variations in the herbs that are used that it is not easy to generalize. If you do try this treatment, find a practitioner with experience in treating IBS.

- *Traditional remedies*—Some sufferers claim relief from a variety of remedies from simple to complex. These might include, for example, certain vitamins (magnesium, vitamin C, B vitamins) or lemon juice or apple cider vinegar with or without hot water. There is no scientific evidence for the benefit of these therapies, but they often have not been tested in this way. Prune juice is an effective laxative for simple constipation (i.e., constipation without pain and bloating), but if you have IBS-related constipation, prune consumption may worsen your symptoms because prunes are high in FODMAPs, particularly sorbitol.

- *Other treatments*—Some sufferers claim that aromatherapy and homeopathy have helped them, but there is no scientific evidence at all that either of these techniques works.

Many people with IBS attempt a combination of strategies for dealing with their individual symptoms and triggers. If a practice seems to help you—and your doctor confirms it is doing you no harm—by all means continue to do it. For a set of research-based dietary guidelines that a majority of IBS sufferers have found helpful and that you can modify to suit your lifestyle and tastes, read on about the low-FODMAP diet.

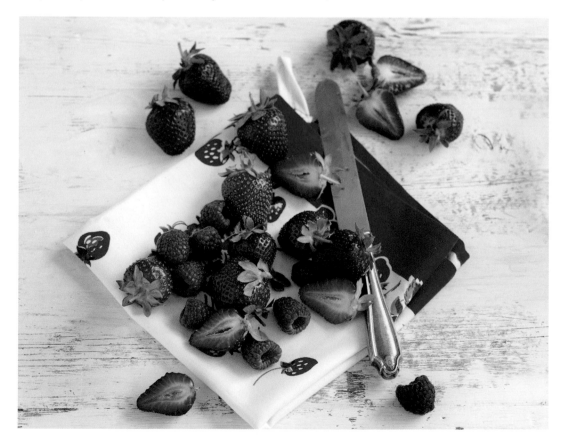

All About the Low-FODMAP Diet

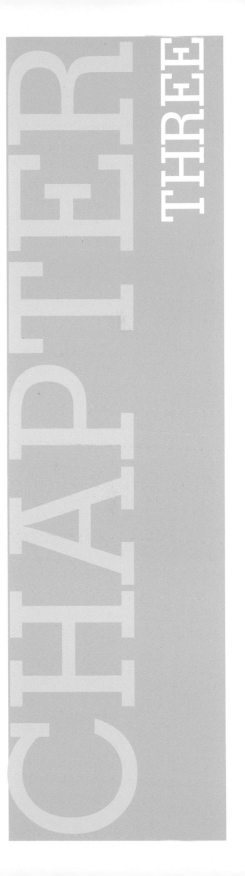

We've seen how the foods we eat can cause the symptoms of irritable bowel syndrome (IBS). Many people who experience IBS have already recognized a strong association between what they eat and the severity of their symptoms.

Many IBS sufferers find changing their diet much more appealing than taking medication. It means they are taking action themselves to relieve their symptoms, and that feeling of empowerment regarding their own health is important. Others, however, prefer to take medication—because it requires less effort on their part and seems like a quick fix. Unfortunately, there is no such thing as a quick fix. Although drugs can relieve *some* symptoms, what is currently available is not very effective overall, and the drugs often come with side effects. Taking medication to manage a lifelong or chronic condition means taking drugs for a long time.

If you have IBS, you are far better off in the long term trying to change your diet.

The low-FODMAP diet has been proven to work for the treatment of IBS symptoms in both the short and long term. Once you know how to follow the diet, it is self-directed and self-empowering, meaning there are no ongoing costs for consultations or drugs. This chapter is all about the low-FODMAP diet—how it works and what it involves.

What are FODMAPs?

As you now know, food intolerances can lead to IBS symptoms (see page 8 for more information on this). Certain food components cause the bowel to distend by drawing in more fluid and rapidly generating gas when they are fermented by bowel bacteria.

The main dietary components that do this are known as fermentable, poorly absorbed short-chain carbohydrates. In other words, they are indigestible sugars that provide fast food for bowel bacteria. As mentioned previously, these sugars have been given the acronym *FODMAP*, which stands for:

Fermentable—rapidly broken down by bacteria in the bowel
Oligosaccharides—fructans and galacto-oligosaccharides (GOS)
Disaccharides—lactose
Monosaccharides—fructose
And
Polyols—sorbitol, mannitol, maltitol, xylitol, polydextrose, and isomalt

Remember, *saccharide* is simply another word for sugar. A monosaccharide has one sugar, a disaccharide has two, an oligosaccharide has a few (less than ten), and a polysaccharide has a large number (more than ten). Polyols are what we call *sugar alcohols*, sugar molecules with an alcohol side-chain. You may have heard of some of these sugars or seen them in ingredients lists, but you don't need to know any more about the chemistry than this.

How do FODMAPs cause symptoms of IBS?

FODMAPs all have the same characteristics:

1. *They are poorly absorbed in the small bowel.* This means that many of these molecules arrive from the

stomach into the small bowel but don't get absorbed, instead passing right through to the colon. This occurs either because they cannot be broken down or they are slow to be absorbed. We all differ in our ability to digest and absorb some FODMAPs: Fructose absorption is slow in all of us but very slow in some; some people do not make enough lactase (the enzyme needed to break down lactose); and the ability to absorb polyols (which are the wrong shape to pass readily through the lining of the small bowel) also varies from person to person. Since none of us can digest fructans and galacto-oligosaccharides (GOS), they are poorly absorbed in everyone.

2. *They are small molecules, consumed in a concentrated dose.* When small, concentrated molecules are poorly absorbed, the body tries to "dilute" them by forcing water into the gastrointestinal tract. Extra fluid in the gastrointestinal tract can cause diarrhea and affect the muscular movement of the gut.

3. *They are "fast food" for the bacteria that live naturally in the large bowel.* The large bowel (and the lower part of the small bowel) naturally contains billions of bacteria. If molecules are not absorbed in the small bowel, they continue the journey to the large bowel. The bacteria that live there see these food molecules as fast food and quickly break them down, which produces hydrogen, carbon dioxide, and methane gases. How quickly the molecules are fermented depends on their chain length: Oligosaccharides and simple sugars are fermented very rapidly compared with fiber, which contains much longer chain molecules, known as polysaccharides.

Multiple types of FODMAPs are usually present in any one meal. Because they all cause distension in the same way once they reach the lower small bowel and colon, their effects are cumulative. This means that the degree of bowel distension can depend upon the total FODMAPs consumed, not just the amount of any individual FODMAP consumed. If someone who cannot digest lactose well and absorbs fructose poorly eats a meal that contains some lactose, some fructans, some polyols, some GOS, and some fructose, the effect on the bowel will be $1 + 1 + 1 + 1 + 1 = 5$ times greater than if they ate the same amount of only one of those FODMAPs. That is why we have to consider all FODMAPs in food when modifying our diet.

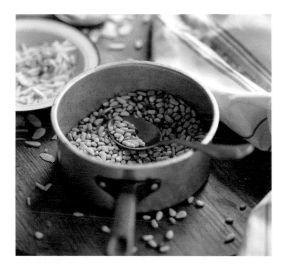

HOW DO WE KNOW THE LOW-FODMAP DIET WORKS?

The first task was to design the low-FODMAP diet. This had never been done before, and it was quite a challenge finding information about the FODMAP content of foods. Once this information was collected, the first version of the diet was developed. The second task was to see if people could understand and follow the diet, and whether it improved symptoms in people with IBS.

We sought a group of IBS sufferers and taught them how to follow the diet. Four out of five found the diet easy to stick to for a long period of time (months and years), and three out of four found that all of their IBS symptoms (pain, bloating, and change in bowel habits) improved markedly. This improvement was greater than we had seen for any drug or other treatment approach. This was only a preliminary experiment, however. It was still necessary to prove that the results were not due to the "placebo effect."

To do this, we rechallenged the patients whose symptoms improved on the low-FODMAP diet, this time with a double-blind, quadruple-arm, randomized, crossover, placebo-controlled rechallenge trial in twenty-five people. This means that we tested twenty-five people by putting them on or off the diet, without them or us knowing whether or not they were taking in FODMAPs.

We supplied these twenty-five people, all of whom had fructose malabsorption, with all their food, which contained no FODMAPs, for twenty-two weeks. In four separate periods of two weeks at a time, the participants added a drink to all of their meals. This drink contained fructans alone, fructose alone, fructans *and* fructose together, or glucose alone (this was the dummy or placebo—most people can absorb glucose without any problems). The drinks all tasted the same, and neither we nor the participants knew which one they were taking. We asked all participants to score the severity of their symptoms every day during the study.

At the end of the study, all the data was locked so that we could make no changes, and then which participant had which drink was revealed to us. Our analysis of the results showed that during those dietary periods when FODMAPs were taken, the participants experienced markedly more symptoms than when only glucose was taken. The fructans alone and fructose alone had similar effects (proving to the skeptics that it is not only fructose that is important), and the fructans *and* fructose had additive effects (i.e., the symptoms were more pronounced when the two sugars were consumed together).

These results have now been published in *Clinical Gastroenterology and Hepatology*, a high-ranking peer-reviewed international medical journal published by the American Gastroenterology Association. This showed that the improvement in these people when they used the low-FODMAP diet was due to the reduction of FODMAPs in the diet. The FODMAP concept was strongly supported.

In subsequent studies, we have supplied food to people with IBS without their knowing whether they were getting low-FODMAP meals or normal-FODMAP meals. These studies showed that the severity of symptoms experienced on a diet of low-FODMAP food was markedly reduced compared to symptoms experienced on a normal- or high-FODMAP diet.

Our clinical experience and other studies have also shown that the diet works for the majority of people with IBS symptoms who do not have fructose malabsorption, and in people with IBS symptoms and inflammatory bowel disease (ulcerative colitis and Crohn's disease; see page 9) who have ongoing gut symptoms despite having their inflammation effectively treated.

We have since looked further into the FODMAP content of various foods and have used this information to refine the low-FODMAP diet. This work is ongoing as more foods continue to be tested for their FODMAP content.

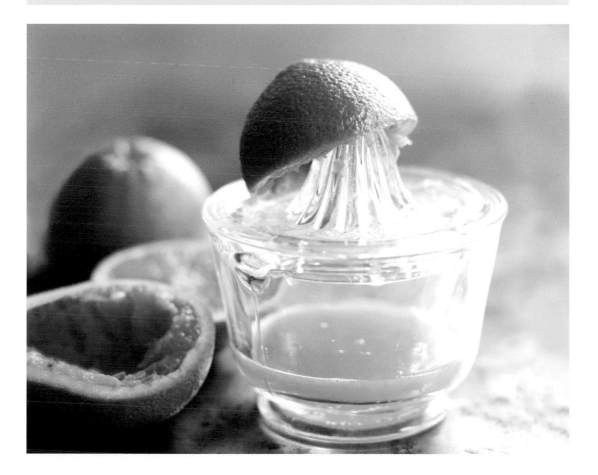

Introducing the FODMAPs

The nature of each type of FODMAP and which foods contain them is outlined below. On pages 44–45, we'll tell you which foods contain a small enough amount of FODMAPs overall to be suitable on the low-FODMAP diet, and on pages 46–47 we'll explain how to test your tolerance for each category of FODMAP.

OLIGOSACCHARIDES

The major types of oligosaccharides found in food that are FODMAPs are fructans and galacto-oligosaccharides (GOS).

Fructans

Fructans are chains of fructose molecules with a glucose molecule at the end. The main dietary sources of fructans include wheat products (breads, cereals, and pasta) and some vegetables, such as onions. Additional sources of fructans are fructo-oligosaccharides (also called oligofructose and FOS) and inulins, which are added to some foods, such as certain yogurts and milk, as a prebiotic (see page 21).

No one is able to digest fructans, and if you have IBS you should minimize your intake of them. Fructans are probably the most common FODMAP to cause symptoms of IBS, probably because most people eat a lot of them. They occur in a wide variety of foods and in large amounts in our food supply.

Foods are considered a problem for sufferers of IBS if they contain more than 0.2 gram of fructans per serving of food for cereals and grains, and 0.3 gram of fructans per serving of food for other foods. The main food sources of fructans are some vegetables and grains, as well as a small number of nuts and fruits.

	HIGH-FRUCTAN FOODS (not suitable)	MODERATE-FRUCTAN FOODS (suitable up to amounts given in parentheses)	LOW-FRUCTAN FOODS (suitable)
FRUITS	nectarines, persimmon, tamarillo, watermelon, white peaches	pomegranate (seeds from ½ small), rambutan (3 whole)	all others
VEGETABLES	artichokes (globe and Jerusalem), garlic, leeks, onions (yellow, red, white, onion powder), scallions (white part), shallots	asparagus (3 spears), beet (½ medium), broccoli (½ cup), Brussels sprouts (½ cup), butternut squash (¼ cup), savoy cabbage (1 cup), fennel (½ cup), green peas (⅓ cup), snow peas (10 pods), sweet corn (½ cob)	alfalfa sprouts, avocados, bamboo shoots, bean shoots, bok choy, bell peppers, carrots, cauliflower, celery, Chinese cabbage, chives, cucumber, eggplant, endive, ginger, green beans, lettuce, mushrooms, olives, parsnips, potatoes, pumpkin, Swiss chard, spinach,

	HIGH-FRUCTAN FOODS (not suitable)	MODERATE-FRUCTAN FOODS (suitable up to amounts given in parentheses)	LOW-FRUCTAN FOODS (suitable)
VEGETABLES (continued)			scallions (green part only), squash (all summer and winter varieties except for butternut squash), rutabaga, sweet potatoes, taro, tomatoes, turnips, watercress, yams, zucchini
CEREALS, GRAINS, AND STARCHES	*wheat-based products*— bread, breakfast cereal, pasta, couscous, noodles, crackers, and cookies in large amounts *rye-based products*— bread and crackers in large amounts *barley-based products*— barley-based products in large amounts (see page 42 for discussion of serving sizes)		arrowroot, buckwheat, cornmeal, cornstarch, millet, oats, popcorn, potatoes, quinoa, rice, sorghum, tapioca
LEGUMES	chickpeas and lentils cooked from dry beans; other beans (e.g., black beans, red kidney beans, borlotti beans, butter beans, navy beans, soybeans, black-eyed peas)	well-rinsed canned chickpeas (up to ¼ cup),* well-rinsed canned red or brown lentils (up to ¼ cup)*	tempeh, tofu
NUTS	pistachios, cashews	almonds (up to 10), hazelnuts (up to 10), one handful of all other nuts and all seeds; 2 tablespoons of nut and seed butters	
DRINKS	chicory-based coffee substitutes		regular tea and coffee, many herbal teas and infusions
FIBER SUPPLEMENTS	wheat bran, inulin (used in some processed foods, e.g., "fiber enriched" products), fructo-oligosaccharides, often in drinks designed as nutritional supplements		chia seeds, flaxseeds, oat bran, psyllium, rice bran

*When canned, these legumes contain smaller amounts of fructans than their dried counterparts. Assess your own tolerance, and include them if you can tolerate them.

Galacto-oligosaccharides (GOS)

Galacto-oligosaccharides (GOS) are chain molecules formed from galactose sugars joined together with a fructose and glucose at the end. Raffinose and stachyose are the most common GOS found in food. They occur in many legumes, such as beans, lentils, and chickpeas.

Like fructans, GOS cannot be digested or absorbed by anybody and they should be avoided if you have IBS. High-GOS foods are those that contain more than 0.2 grams per serving.

Note that some people can tolerate up to ¼ cup of well-rinsed canned lentils or chickpeas better than dry legumes that have been soaked and cooked. Assess your own tolerance.

HIGH-GOS FOODS	
LEGUMES	beans (e.g., kidney, baked, black, cannellini, great northern, pinto, navy, lima, butter, adzuki, soy, mung, and fava beans), chickpeas, lentils

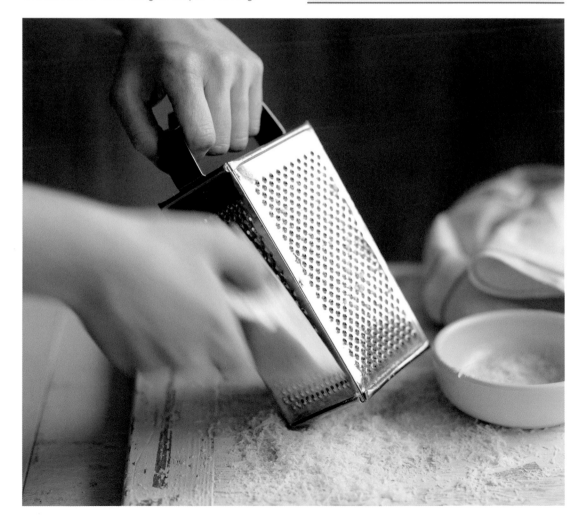

DISACCHARIDES

Only one disaccharide can potentially act as a FODMAP in food—lactose.

Lactose

Lactose is a double sugar that occurs naturally in all animal milks, including milk from cows, sheep, and goats. Made up of two digestible sugars called glucose and galactose, it is broken down in the small bowel into its component sugars by an enzyme called lactase. Lactose-intolerant people, however, have low levels of lactase and can therefore only break down a very small amount of the lactose they consume. Such people may benefit from reducing their lactose intake as part of the low-FODMAP diet. Experience has shown that reducing lactose intake alone (without also reducing intake of the other FODMAPs) is not very effective at minimizing IBS symptoms.

Most people who are lactase-deficient, however, still produce a small amount of the lactase enzyme and do not need to remove lactase completely from their diet.

A lactose-free diet is *not* a dairy-free diet. Lactose is present in varying amounts in milk and milk products such as yogurt, kefir, ice cream, pudding and other desserts, and soft, unripened cheeses (such as cottage, ricotta, and cream cheeses). Cream contains a minimal amount of lactose, and hard and ripened cheeses (such as Cheddar, Parmesan, Camembert, Edam, Gouda, blue, and mozzarella) and butter are virtually lactose-free.

Most people with lactose malabsorption can handle up to 4 grams of lactose per serving of food without experiencing problems.

A thin spread of butter or margarine and small amounts of milk in tea and coffee, chocolate, cakes, and cookies may be tolerated, whereas a full glass of milk would cause symptoms. If you are lactase-deficient, you should restrict lactose-containing foods based on your own degree of sensitivity.

LACTOSE CONTENT OF COMMON FOODS AND DRINKS

FOOD OR BEVERAGE (serving size)	LACTOSE (grams)
whole milk (1 cup)	16
low-fat milk (1 cup)	15
skim milk (1 cup)	13
evaporated milk (½ cup)	13
cottage cheese (½ cup)	8
low-fat yogurt (6 ounces)	6
whole milk yogurt (6 ounces)	6
cheesecake (1 small slice)	6
milk chocolate (2 ounces)	6
ice cream (2 scoops)	4
béchamel (white sauce) (2 tablespoons)	2
cake (1 small slice)	1
full-fat cream cheese (1 tablespoon)	1
sour cream (1 tablespoon)	0.5
cream (1 tablespoon)	0.4
butter (1 tablespoon)	0.1
cheese (1 ounce)	0.1

High-lactose foods contain more than 4 grams of lactose per serving, moderate-lactose foods contain 1 to 4 grams of lactose per serving, and low-lactose foods contain less than 1 gram per serving. High-lactose foods may be safely consumed in small quantities, as indicated in the following table.

HIGH-LACTOSE FOODS AND ALTERNATIVES

	HIGH-LACTOSE FOODS	MODERATE-LACTOSE FOODS (suitable up to amounts given in parentheses)	LOW-LACTOSE FOODS AND ALLOWABLE SERVINGS OF HIGH-LACTOSE FOODS
MILK	whole, low-fat, and skim cow's, goat's, or sheep's milk	*small quantities*—regular milk in tea and coffee	whole, low-fat, and skim lactose-free milk; soy milk (choose varieties made from soybean extract, *not* whole soybeans); rice, oat, almond, and quinoa milks (choose calcium-fortified)
MILK PRODUCTS	ice cream, dairy-based desserts, pudding, milk powder (also called "milk solids" or "milk solids non-fat"), evaporated milk, sweetened condensed milk	*small quantities*—regular milk or milk powder in cakes, cookies, and snacks (e.g., milk chocolate), cream (up to ⅓ cup), butter	soy or almond ice cream (choose calcium-fortified), lactose-free cream
YOGURT	full-fat, low-fat, and skim cow's, sheep's and goat's yogurt		almond, soy,* or rice yogurts (without inulin); lactose-free yogurts
CHEESE	soft cheeses (e.g., cottage cheese, cream cheese, crème fraîche, mascarpone, ricotta)		hard, formed, and ripened cheeses (blue, Brie, Cheddar, Colby, Edam, Emmental, feta, Gorgonzola, Gouda, Gruyère, Havarti, Monterey Jack, mozzarella, Neufchâtel, Parmesan, pecorino, provolone, Raclette, Stilton, Swiss, Taleggio), soy cheese;* soft cheeses (up to 2 ounces)

*These contain GOS and/or fructans, but in small amounts as part of a recipe do not cause IBS symptoms in most people. You should assess your own tolerance.

MONOSACCHARIDES

The only important monosaccharide that can potentially act as a FODMAP in food is fructose.

Fructose

Fructose, a single sugar, is often referred to as the "fruit sugar." It is found in every fruit, in honey, and in high-fructose corn syrup. It is a component of table sugar (also called sucrose or cane sugar) and is also found in some vegetables (e.g., sugar snap peas) and grains (e.g., wheat).

When fructose occurs with glucose, it is well absorbed because it is "piggybacked" across the bowel lining by the glucose. If fructose is found in higher concentrations than glucose (a situation we call *excess fructose*), however, its absorption is slower. When it is incomplete, it is called *fructose malabsorption*. This is not an illness or a condition. It is just a part of a person's physiology: Some people are not well equipped to absorb excess fructose, while others are. About one in three people has fructose malabsorption. It is not more common in people with IBS.

If you have fructose malabsorption, there is no need to avoid fructose (or fruit) completely. As long as the fructose in a food is balanced with glucose, or there is more glucose than fructose, you can eat moderate amounts without experiencing IBS symptoms. The table below demonstrates this concept.

Foods are considered a problem for IBS sufferers if they contain more than 0.2 gram fructose in excess of glucose per serving. Foods and beverages with 0.1 to 0.2 gram more fructose than glucose per serving do not usually induce symptoms. The main food sources of excess fructose are fruits.

All good things should be enjoyed in moderation. The gut can be overloaded by lots of fructose even if glucose is in balance with the fructose. So you should not only choose fruits in which fructose and glucose are in balance, but also limit the amount of such fruit you eat in one sitting. The total fruit quantity should be approximately equal to the size of an average orange. You can enjoy several servings of fruit per day, but ensure they are spread out, with at least two hours between.

CALCULATING THE FREE-FRUCTOSE CONTENT OF FOODS

FOOD	FRUCTOSE (per 100 grams)	GLUCOSE (per 100 grams)	EXCESS FREE FRUCTOSE (column 2 minus column 3)	CONCLUSION
honey	40	30	10	problem
mango	2	1.5	0.5	problem
kiwi	**4**	**4**	**0**	**suitable**

An acceptable single fruit intake could be one of the following:

- 1 whole banana or orange
- 2 kiwi or tangerines
- 1 small slice of melon or pineapple
- ⅓ to ½ cup (80 to 120 ml) of any suitable 100 percent fruit juice (e.g. orange juice, *not* apple or pear juice)
- 1 small handful of berries or grapes
- A very small amount of suitable dried fruit (e.g., 10 dried banana chips, ¼ cup/20 g unsweetened shredded coconut)
- 3 tablespoons tomato paste or fruit-based sauce or chutney, unsweetened or with suitable sweeteners

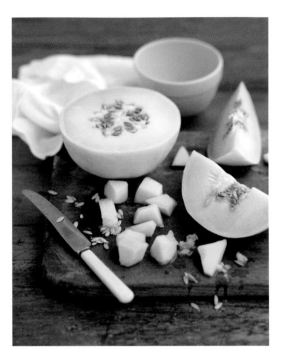

	FOODS CONTAINING EXCESS FREE FRUCTOSE (not suitable)	LOW-FRUCTOSE OR BALANCED FOODS
FRUITS	apples, Asian pears, boysenberries, cherries, figs, mangoes, pears, tamarillo, watermelon	*in small quantities*—apricots, avocados, bananas, blackberries, blueberries, cranberries, durian, grapefruit, grapes, honeydew melon, kiwi, kumquats, lemons, limes, longans, oranges, nectarines, oranges, passion fruit, papaya, peaches, pineapple, plums, raspberries, rhubarb, cantaloupe, star fruit, strawberries, tangelos, tangerines, tomatoes
VEGETABLES	asparagus, artichokes, sugar snap peas	all others
SWEETENERS AND CONDIMENTS	agave nectar, high-fructose corn syrup, fructose, fruit juice concentrate, honey	*in moderation*—sucrose (table sugar, cane sugar), including superfine sugar, confectioners' sugar, brown sugar, raw sugar; glucose; maple syrup, molasses, rice syrup; yeast extract spreads (e.g., Marmite); peanut butter, other nut butters except cashew butter; chocolate-nut spreads (e.g., Nutella); jam and marmalade in small quantities (limit intake of "100 percent fruit spreads," which are often sweetened with pear juice)

POLYOLS

Polyols, also called sugar alcohols, are often given names that end in "ol" and include sorbitol, mannitol, maltitol, xylitol, polydextrose, and isomalt. Polyols occur naturally in some fruits and vegetables. They are often used in food manufacturing as humectants (water-binding agents) and artificial sweeteners—particularly in "sugar-free" chewing gums, mints, and candy. When polyols are used as an artificial sweetener, the packaging will state "Excess consumption may have a laxative effect." Foods are considered a problem

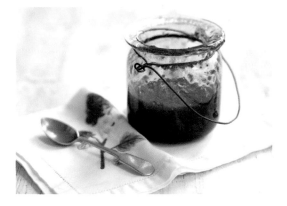

for IBS sufferers if they contain more than 0.5 gram total polyols per serving.

	HIGH-POLYOL FOODS (not suitable)	MODERATE-POLYOL FOODS (suitable up to the amounts listed in parentheses)	LOW-POLYOL FOODS (suitable)
FRUITS	apples, apricots, Asian pears, blackberries, nectarines, peaches, pears, plums, prunes, watermelon	cherries (3), longans (10), lychee (5)	bananas, blueberries, cranberries, durian, grapefruit, grapes, honeydew melon, kiwi, lemons, limes, mangoes, oranges, passion fruit, papaya, pineapple, raspberries, rhubarb, cantaloupe, star fruit, strawberries, tangelos, tangerines
VEGETABLES	cauliflower, mushrooms, snow peas	avocado (¼), celery (1 stalk), sweet potato (½ cup)	all others
"DIET," "SUGAR-FREE," OR "LOW-CARB" FOODS	gums, mints, candy, desserts, and other products containing polyol additives as artificial sweeteners (see "Additives," below); foods with the warning "Excess consumption may have a laxative effect."		chewing gum sweetened with sugar (sucrose), sugar-sweetened mints and candy
ADDITIVES	sorbitol, mannitol, maltitol, xylitol, polydextrose, isomalt		aspartame, saccharine, stevia

HOW DO WE KNOW WHAT FODMAPS DO IN THE BOWEL?

It is easy to show that the FODMAPs are fast food for bacteria, although we don't suggest you try it at home. In the lab, we take feces, mix it up, and add any of the FODMAPs. The bacteria in the feces rapidly ferment the FODMAP added. We know this because as the FODMAP disappears, gas is produced and the feces becomes more acidic (because acids are produced during fermentation).

Research in studies with people who have had an ileostomy (their large bowel has been removed and the contents of their small bowel empty directly into a bag) has shown that FODMAPs are poorly absorbed from the small bowel. Nearly all the FODMAPs consumed in food can be detected in the matter that empties from the ileostomy.

Research at Monash University in Melbourne, Australia, in people who have had an ileostomy has shown that FODMAPs draw water into the bowel. The researchers fed these people a high-FODMAP diet and then a low-FODMAP diet, or vice versa.

The amount of liquid matter that was emptied into the ileostomy bag was much greater when they ate a high-FODMAP diet. This proved that FODMAPs increase the amount of liquid in the bowel, which can in turn cause diarrhea (see pages 13–14). One way to reduce diarrhea, then, is to reduce the intake of FODMAPs in the diet.

We can prove that a high-FODMAP diet increases gas production by measuring how much hydrogen is present in the breath of people who have eaten a diet containing the same amount of fiber and starch, but either a lot of or only a few FODMAPs. Hydrogen in the breath comes from gases produced by bacteria in the bowel, and fermentation of carbohydrates by bacteria in the bowel is the only way that hydrogen is produced in the body. We measured the hydrogen in the breath of healthy volunteers and people with IBS. The breath of people in both groups who ate a high-FODMAP diet had increased hydrogen levels compared with those who ate a low-FODMAP diet.

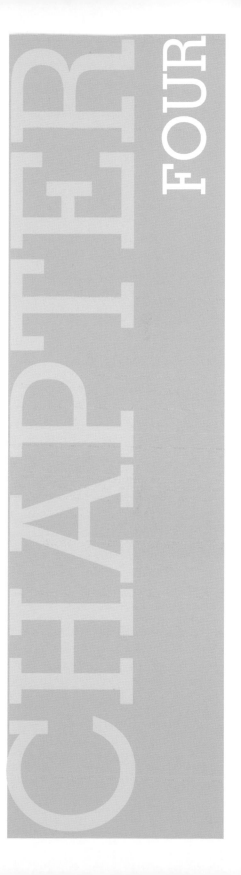

Implementing the Low-FODMAP Diet

If you've been diagnosed with IBS, or you've experienced bloating and abdominal discomfort with or without a change in your bowel habits, or you and/or your doctor believe you should follow the low-FODMAP diet for another reason, your first step should be to contact a registered dietitian who specializes in gastrointestinal nutrition.

That is not to say that the low-FODMAP diet is difficult to manage, but it will mean significant diet and lifestyle changes. You will have to learn about your condition, which foods are suitable, and what will happen if you cease following the diet.

Where do I start?

To keep your symptoms under control, we recommend that you follow the low-FODMAP diet strictly by avoiding *all* FODMAPs for at least two months. If your symptoms have improved after this time, it is recommended to gradually reintroduce one FODMAP group at a time to see if you tolerate it. This is easier to do with the help of a registered dietitian, who will review your symptoms and suggest the best approach, but for more on how to do it yourself and menu plans, see pages 46–48 and 64–75. For advice for starting the diet alongside other special dietary needs, see pages 55–60.

Before you start the low-FODMAP diet, you may want to have a breath hydrogen test (see page 40), to check whether you have fructose or lactose malabsorption or both. If you discover that you don't have either, you will be able to include lactose and fructose in your low-FODMAP diet, although a negative breath test for fructose and lactose does not mean you won't benefit from restricting the other

remaining FODMAPs. If you decide not to have a breath test, we recommend you avoid *all* FODMAPs for the initial two months.

You may find aspects of the low-FODMAP diet overwhelming at first. You will have to ask yourself these questions each morning: Where am I going to be today? Do I need to take food with me? Should I eat before I go? Will there be something there that I can eat? If you require a special diet, it can start to dictate your thoughts, and some people cope with this better than others. If you are having trouble adjusting, seek counseling or other help.

Here are some other important points to bear in mind when tailoring the low-FODMAP diet to your needs:

- *Consider all the FODMAP groups.* They all have the potential to cause bowel distension and other IBS symptoms.
- *No one can absorb fructans, GOS, or polyols well.* This means you should always avoid them when first implementing the low-FODMAP diet.
- *Only some people have lactose or fructose malabsorption.* A breath hydrogen test will tell you whether or not you need to limit lactose or excess fructose in your diet.
- *Some FODMAPs cause more trouble in some people than others.* This depends on the proportions of each FODMAP in their diet, how well or poorly they absorb fructose and lactose, and how sensitive they are to each FODMAP, which could be related to which bacteria they have in their bowel. You'll learn which FODMAPs give you the most trouble through a combination of clinical tests and trial in your diet (see pages 46–47).

REGISTERED DIETITIANS

The low-FODMAP diet was designed to be taught by a registered dietitian, preferably one knowledgeable about the low-FODMAP diet rather than one just following a food chart and instruction sheet. Although this book is a great resource for anyone following the low-FODMAP diet, we also strongly recommend that you consult with a registered dietitian. Here are a few good reasons to seek out expert help before starting the low-FODMAP diet:

- The diet has many guidelines, and to succeed, it must be incorporated into your own individual eating style and food choices. A registered dietitian specializing in gastrointestinal nutrition will look at your eating patterns and preferences, identify the main culprits in your diet, and recommend alternatives to those foods you tend to eat that are high in FODMAPs.
- The registered dietitian will ensure that your individualized low-FODMAP diet plan has plenty of variety, so that it is both interesting to eat and nutritionally adequate. A registered dietitian will ensure you are not cutting out more foods than is necessary for symptom relief.
- Two keys to the success of the low-FODMAP diet are understanding its underlying basis and sticking to it. A nutrition expert can answer your questions about the diet, help you with unfamiliar foods and situations, and help you keep your diet on track.
- The registered dietitian will provide high-quality reference material for you, including food lists, cookbooks, and shopping guides.

PREPARE FOR YOUR FIRST VISIT

Before your first visit, let the registered dietitian know you would like to try the low-FODMAP diet. The dietitian will want to know your patterns of eating and the food choices you make. This can be done at the consultation, but obtaining information takes some time and eats into the consultation time. Instead, we recommend you keep a seven-day food and symptom diary. Make sure to continue your normal food intake patterns. Many people change their eating habits when they are requested to record what they eat! Your diary should include all meals, snacks, and beverages you ate during the week, as well as the timing, severity, and type of symptoms you felt. A food diary reflecting your usual habits is essential for identifying potential triggers and focusing the discussion on things that are relevant to you. This is what we call "individualizing" therapy and advice. To track your food intake and corresponding symptoms, photocopy and fill in the sample food and symptom diary on pages 258–259. Alternatively, you can try one of the food and symptom diary services available online or on your smartphone.

REGISTERED DIETITIANS WITH EXPERTISE IN THE LOW-FODMAP DIET

It is recommended that you consult with your local gastroenterologist or general practitioner. Additional resources for finding a registered dietitian appear on page 255.

BREATH HYDROGEN TESTS

Breath hydrogen tests can be useful to help plan a low-FODMAP diet.

Hydrogen is a gas that is produced by bacteria in the bowel when they ferment carbohydrates. Some of the hydrogen produced is absorbed across the lining of the large bowel into the bloodstream.

The bloodstream then transports it to the lungs, where it is breathed out. Bacterial fermentation in the bowel is the *only* source of hydrogen gas in the breath. The same applies to the gas methane—in about 10 percent of the population, the bacteria in the large bowel make methane rather than hydrogen. In a breath hydrogen test, we use a special instrument to measure the amount of hydrogen and methane gases exhaled from the lungs.

If you do the test, you will be asked to minimize your intake of fiber and FODMAPs in food for twenty-four hours beforehand so that there will be little, if any, hydrogen in the breath. You will also have to fast for several hours before the test. You will be asked to breathe into a bag or a handheld machine so that your breath sample can be taken. You will then be asked to drink a solution of a test sugar dissolved in water, and breath samples will be taken every fifteen to twenty minutes for up to four hours.

Three sugars—lactulose, fructose, and lactose—are usually tested. Lactulose cannot be digested or absorbed and is used to determine how vigorously your bacteria produce hydrogen and how fast the sugar travels out of the stomach and down the small intestine. Fructose and lactose are then tested. If your gut symptoms are triggered during or after the test, they will be noted down by the technician.

Any rise in the amount of hydrogen (or methane) in your breath after the sugar drink will mean that the sugar is being fermented by bacteria in your bowel and, therefore, that it is not completely absorbed. If fructose or lactose is completely absorbed (i.e., there is no rise in breath hydrogen), there is little need to restrict them in your diet. If your breath hydrogen does rise after you ingest fructose or lactose, then you should restrict them as part of your low-FODMAP diet.

For more information on breath hydrogen tests and their interpretation, see this book's website, www.thelowfodmapdiet.com.

How important is it to have breath hydrogen testing? The results of such tests will

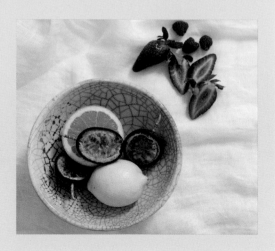

not determine whether the low-FODMAP diet is suitable for you. They just indicate that lactose and excess fructose can be absorbed well or not. Knowing that lactose or excess fructose malabsorption is not a problem for you indicates that your diet need not restrict lactose or fructose. However, this information can also be gained by assessing your response to challenging with fructose-rich or lactose-rich foods (see pages 46–47). Thus, getting a breath test is not an essential part of following the diet.

Still, many doctors, dietitians, and patients prefer to have breath testing prior to starting the diet. Ask your doctor or dietitian if you're interested in having these tests run.

A low-FODMAP diet Q&A

Which FODMAPs should I avoid?
When you start the low-FODMAP diet, you should avoid *all* FODMAPs—fructans, GOS, lactose, excess fructose, and polyols. If you know you can completely absorb fructose, however, you need not restrict your excess fructose intake, and if you know you can completely absorb lactose, you need not restrict your lactose intake.

How much fruit can I eat at one sitting, and how do I limit my fructose load?
You should eat no more than one serving of suitable fruits (see page 45) per meal or sitting. One serving is usually one cup of cut-up fruit or one whole piece of fruit, such as one orange or banana. You can enjoy many fruit servings each day, but you should allow two to three hours between each serving.

Can I eat "table sugar"?
Table sugar (also called sucrose or cane sugar) should not cause symptoms if eaten in moderation. Sucrose is a double sugar made up of one part glucose and one part fructose.

How do I balance my glucose and fructose intake?
If you need to avoid excess fructose, then consuming glucose at the same time as fructose could reduce the severity of your symptoms. You should be aware, however, that this strategy is not recommended if you have diabetes. Glucose sources include glucose powders and tablets, which are available in the sports-drink section of the supermarket and some health-food stores. How much glucose you need to consume with an excess of fructose will depend on how much of the food you are eating and what other foods you have recently consumed or are consuming at the same time. The best way is to use trial and error to establish how much glucose you require to remain free of IBS symptoms while consuming a food that has an excess of fructose. This strategy is unlikely to help when eating foods with excess fructose *and* other FODMAPS.

What about fats and protein foods?
Fats and oils do not contain FODMAPs, nor do animal-based protein foods, such as meat, fish, chicken, and eggs. However, plant-based protein foods such as legumes do contain FODMAPs, and you may need to restrict your

intake of these foods. FODMAPs typically occur in carbohydrate-based foods.

How do I avoid FODMAPs if I'm a vegetarian? What if I'm a vegan?

Vegetarians often consume large amounts of legumes as an important source of protein. Tofu and tempeh are low in FODMAPs, but legumes generally contain GOS and fructans. As there is a risk that your vegetarian or vegan diet will become nutritionally inadequate if you cut out legumes, a registered dietitian experienced in the low-FODMAP diet may advise you to allow a certain amount of legumes in your diet but to exclude all other food sources of FODMAPs. The best approach will depend on your individual tolerance. For more tips, see page 55.

Must I really avoid wheat products?

If you follow the low-FODMAP diet, you must avoid eating wheat, rye, and barley in large quantities. This means you should avoid breads, cereals, pasta, and cookies, but you can still enjoy such things as a bread-crumb coating on fried chicken or cookie pieces in ice cream. A registered dietitian knowledgeable about the low-FODMAP diet can help assess your individual intolerance to wheat and rye products. The table on the facing page lists common wheat-based products and suitable alternatives.

Some people may tolerate small amounts of 100 percent spelt bread, but not other spelt products (e.g., pasta and breakfast cereals, which are high in FODMAPs). Once you have been on the low-FODMAP diet for several weeks and your symptoms have improved, it might be worth trying small amounts of 100 percent spelt bread to assess your own tolerance.

One bonus of a reduced-wheat diet is that you consume a greater variety of other grains, which means you can obtain a greater range of nutrients. An enormous variety of specialty gluten-free (and so free of wheat, barley, and rye) foods is now available, including delicious pasta, baking mixes, breakfast cereals, breads, cookies, and snack bars. You will find specialty gluten-free alternatives in the health-food aisle of your supermarket and in health-food stores. It's important to feel confident reading and interpreting food ingredient labels, and further guidance on this is provided on page 78.

Do I really need to avoid onions and garlic?

Onion is one of the greatest contributors to IBS symptoms. We recommend that you strictly avoid onion for at least two months. This means not only cooking without onion (all varieties, plus leeks, shallots, and the white part of scallions) but also avoiding packaged foods that contain onion ingredients, such as onion powder in soups and stocks. You may find that you can reintroduce onion into your diet, but this will probably be only in very small amounts. If you cook with onion but leave it on your plate, this will only *reduce* the fructan load rather than remove it, since fructans can leach out of the onion into the other ingredients during cooking. Garlic also contains fructans, though if you like the flavor, one to two cloves per recipe (which serves four to six people) can often be tolerated by IBS sufferers. An even better way to enjoy the taste of garlic without the fructans is to use garlic-infused oil.

SUGGESTED ALTERNATIVES TO WHEAT-BASED FOODS

	WHEAT-BASED VARIETIES	SUGGESTED ALTERNATIVES
BREAD	white, whole wheat, multigrain, and sourdough breads, pita bread, many "rye breads"	corn tortillas, gluten-free bread,* gluten-free flatbread,* 100% spelt bread (for some people)
PASTA, NOODLES, AND GRAINS	regular pasta, spelt pasta, most instant noodles, egg noodles, udon, gnocchi, bulgur, farro	gluten-free pasta,* glass (mungbean) noodles, rice noodles (vermicelli), wheat-free soba (buckwheat) noodles
BREAKFAST CEREALS	most are made from wheat and may also contain excess dried fruit or be sweetened with fruit juice	many gluten-free breakfast cereals, cornflakes, wheat-free fruit-free muesli, oatmeal, quinoa flakes, rice flakes, rice puffs
CRACKERS	wheat-based varieties, water crackers	corn thins, gluten-free crackers, gluten-free crispbread (such as buckwheat), rice cakes or crackers (but check for onion powder)
CAKES AND BAKED GOODS	most are made from wheat	flourless cakes, gluten-free cakes,* gluten-free baking mixes*
COOKIES	wheat-based varieties	almond macaroons, gluten-free cookies*
PASTRY AND BREAD CRUMBS	made with wheat flour	gluten-free pastry mixes,* cornflake crumbs, gluten-free bread crumbs* (although wheat-based crumbs can usually be tolerated in small amounts)
OTHER CEREAL PRODUCTS	semolina, couscous, bulgur	buckwheat, chestnut, chia seeds, corn, millet, polenta, potatoes, quinoa, rice, sago, sorghum, tapioca, and their flours

*Gluten-free baked goods may contain ingredients unsuited to the low-FODMAP diet, such as fruit juice concentrate as a sweetener or high-FODMAP flours. If high-FODMAP foods are high on the ingredients list, the food should be avoided; however, a food including these ingredients lower on the list (i.e., in small quantities) may be tolerated. Check the ingredients list and assess your own tolerance.

Are there other ways to tackle lactose malabsorption?

If you have lactose malabsorption, you can buy lactase enzyme in tablets in pharmacies and some health-food stores. The enzyme will break down the lactose in lactose-containing foods and beverages so that you can absorb it. This may help enhance variety in your diet and make it easier for you when eating away from home. Take lactase tablets at the same time as the lactose-containing food or drink (refer to the package instructions for how many to take).

How do I know which foods I can eat?

The table on the following pages summarizes foods that contain FODMAPs and suitable alternatives.

FODMAP-CONTAINING FOODS AND SUITABLE ALTERNATIVES

	HIGH-FODMAP VARIETIES	LOW-FODMAP ALTERNATIVES
FLOURS AND GRAINS (INCLUDING LEGUME PRODUCTS)	barley, bulgur, chickpea flour (besan),* couscous, durum, Kamut®, lentil flour,* multigrain flour, pea flour,* rye, semolina, soy flour,* triticale, wheat bran, wheat flour, wheat germ	arrowroot, buckwheat flour, cornmeal, cornstarch, gluten-free flour blends,** glutinous rice, ground rice, malt, millet, oat bran, oatmeal, polenta, popcorn, potato flour, quinoa, rice (brown, white), rice bran, rice flour, sago, sorghum, tapioca, wild rice
CEREALS	wheat-based and mixed-grain breakfast cereals, muesli	baby rice cereal, cream of buckwheat, rice- or corn-based breakfast cereals, oatmeal, wheat-free, fruit-free muesli
PASTA AND NOODLES	noodles, pasta, spaetzle, gnocchi	glass (mungbean) noodles, rice noodles, rice vermicelli, 100% buckwheat soba noodles, gluten-free pasta
BREADS, COOKIES, AND CAKES	breads (including sourdough), bread crumbs, cookies, cakes, croissants, muffins, and pastries containing wheat and rye	gluten-free breads,** corn tortillas and taco shells, plain rice cakes and crackers, gluten-free cookies,** gluten-free cakes and pastries**
DAIRY FOODS AND ALTERNATIVES	regular milk, ice cream, soft cheeses (in amounts greater than ½ cup), yogurt	lactose-free milk; most lactose-free yogurts and kefir; lactose-free ice cream; calcium-fortified soy,† rice, oat, and quinoa milks, yogurts, and ice creams; butter and margarine; hard and ripened cheeses, including Brie and Camembert; gelato and sorbets made from suitable fruits and sweeteners; moderate servings of cream (less than ½ cup)
MEAT AND VEGETARIAN PROTEIN SOURCES	certain sausages (check for onion and dehydrated vegetable powders)	bacon, eggs, fish, poultry, plain red meat, tempeh, tofu
NUTS AND SEEDS	pistachios and cashews	all other nuts and seeds; nut and seed butters not made from pistachios or cashews (no more than a handful of nuts and seeds or 2 tablespoons of nut or seed butters in a meal)

*These contain GOS and/or fructans, but in small amounts as part of a recipe, they do not cause IBS symptoms in most people. You should assess your own tolerance.

**Gluten-free baked goods may contain ingredients unsuited to the low-FODMAP diet, such as fruit juice concentrate as a sweetener or high-FODMAP flours. If high-FODMAP foods are high on the ingredients list, the food should be avoided; however, a food including these ingredients lower on the list (i.e., in small quantities) may be tolerated. Check the ingredients list and assess your own tolerance.

†Soy milks made from soybean *extract* (not whole soybeans) are well tolerated.

	HIGH-FODMAP VARIETIES	LOW-FODMAP ALTERNATIVES
VEGETABLES	artichokes (globe and Jerusalem), asparagus, cauliflower, garlic, leeks, mushrooms, onions (yellow, red, white, onion powder), scallions (white part), shallots, snow peas, sugar snap peas	alfalfa sprouts, bamboo shoots, bean sprouts, bell pepper, bok choy, broccoli, carrot, chayote, Chinese cabbage, cucumber, eggplant, green beans, lettuce (butter, iceberg, romaine), olives, parsnip, potatoes, pumpkin, rutabagas, Swiss chard, spinach, scallion (green part only), squash (all tested varieties except butternut squash—note that not all have been tested), taro, turnips, watercress, yams, zucchini
FRUITS	apples, apricots, Asian pears, blackberries, boysenberries, cherries, figs, mangoes, nectarines, peaches, pears, persimmon, plums, prunes, tamarillo, watermelon, white peaches	bananas, blueberries, cantaloupe, cranberries, durian, grapefruit, grapes, honeydew melon, kiwi, lemons, limes, mandarin oranges, oranges, passion fruit, papaya, raspberries, star fruit, strawberries, tangelos, tangerines, tomatoes
SPREADS AND CONDIMENTS	most commercial relishes, chutneys, onion-containing gravies, stock and bouillon cubes, dressings, and sauces	jam, marmalade, mayonnaise, mustard, soy sauce, garlic-free sweet chili sauce or hot sauce, tamari, vinegar
SWEETENERS	agave nectar, honey, high-fructose corn syrup, corn syrup solids, fructose, fruit juice concentrate; sorbitol, mannitol, maltitol, xylitol	sucrose (table sugar, cane sugar), including superfine sugar, confectioners' sugar, brown sugar, raw sugar; glucose; maple syrup, molasses, rice syrup; artificial sweeteners not ending in "ol" (e.g., aspartame, saccharine, and stevia)
BEVERAGES	apple, pear, and mango juices; other fruit juices in amounts greater than ½ cup; chicory-based coffee substitutes	water, mineral water, soda water, sugar-sweetened soft drinks, tonic water, fruit juice (safe fruits only, ½ cup (125 ml) per serving), most teas, coffee, most alcohol (see pages 52–53)
FATS AND OILS	applesauce as oil replacer in low-fat baked goods	vegetable oils, butter, ghee, lard, drippings, margarine, garlic-infused oil as an onion and garlic substitute
OTHERS		baking powder, baking soda, cocoa, coconut, gelatin, salt, xanthan gum, fresh and dried herbs and spices (besides garlic and onion powder; see page 78), chives, ginger

Reintroducing the FODMAPs one at a time

All FODMAPs can cause IBS symptoms, and if they are eaten together, their effect is cumulative. Any meal is likely to contain a variety of foods and, therefore, a complex mixture of carbohydrates, which includes FODMAPs. The low-FODMAP diet aims to reduce the intake of *all* FODMAPs so that IBS symptoms are reduced as much as possible.

While all FODMAPs are potential triggers for IBS symptoms, which FODMAP has the greatest effect on you will depend on how much and how often you consume foods that contain them. In many cultures, fructose and fructans are the most widespread and frequently eaten FODMAPs. Lactose, GOS, and polyol intake can vary significantly. Intake can also vary seasonally: Sorbitol intake is likely to be higher in summer when stone fruits are in abundance. Indian and Mexican cuisines, which are based largely on lentils and beans, will have a higher GOS content.

Once you have followed the low-FODMAP diet for two months and have seen an improvement in your symptoms, you can reintroduce the FODMAPs, one at a time, to determine which contribute to your symptoms and how much of each you can tolerate. This process is called a food challenge. Here are some guidelines for FODMAP food challenges:

1. Test only one FODMAP subgroup at a time. (Use the suggestions in the flowchart on the opposite page.)
2. Choose an amount of food that reflects a normal portion size. You will gain no useful information about your tolerance of a FODMAP group if you challenge yourself with a very large—or unreasonably small—intake in your trial dose. Any food consumed in excessive amounts is likely to induce symptoms.
3. Where possible, choose a food that contains only one type of FODMAP, to enable a more accurate interpretation of your response.
4. Continue to restrict *all* other FODMAPs until your tolerance (or intolerance) is confirmed.
5. Maintain a consistent intake of caffeine and alcohol, or of any other foods you know are a problem for you.
6. Challenge with one FODMAP per week.
7. Eat the challenge food at least twice during the test week (or until symptoms are triggered).

Monitor your symptom response.

If you don't get symptoms:

- Increase the number of foods that contain the FODMAP you are testing, and assess your response
- *Or* maintain the amount and type of food you have tested, and then undertake the next FODMAP challenge.

If you do get symptoms:

- Wait until you are symptom free, then reduce the serving size to half and challenge again
- *Or* assume the FODMAP is a problem for you. It is recommended to continue to restrict the FODMAP and to try the suggestions that follow.

- ➤ Try another food from within the same FODMAP group to confirm the result of the challenge.
- ➤ The dose of FODMAPs is vital when challenging foods. We suggest you halve the amount of food and try again when you are symptom free. It is unlikely you will have to omit the FODMAP completely.
- ➤ We encourage you to challenge again in the future, as your sensitivity to FODMAPs may change over time.

A suggested order, type, and quantity of food for the reintroduction of each FODMAP subgroup appear in the below flowchart. The order is a guide only—choose an order that works for you.

FODMAP REINTRODUCTION PLAN

POLYOLS	**sorbitol**—2 medium fresh apricots (*or* 4 dried apricot halves) **mannitol**—½ cup mushrooms

⬇

LACTOSE	½ to 1 cup milk *or* 6 ounces yogurt

⬇

FRUCTOSE	½ mango *or* 1 teaspoon honey

⬇

FRUCTANS	2 slices wheat bread *or* 1 clove garlic, then build up to testing ¼ onion (this should be tested last as onions have a very high fructan content)

⬇

GALACTO-OLIGOSACCHARIDES	½ cup lentils, kidney beans, baked beans, *or* chickpeas

What if the low-FODMAP diet doesn't work for me?

Although the low-FODMAP diet is very effective, it is not a panacea: For about one in four people it has little, if any, effect on IBS symptoms, although this is often because they are not being absolutely strict about following the diet. You must be dedicated to the diet; being selective about what you restrict won't work. However, for a small proportion of IBS sufferers, diet itself is not a factor. Some, for instance, swallow too much air, or their gut has trouble handling even the normal amount of air they swallow. Such people need to avoid carbonated beverages and drinking liquids too quickly. Many can benefit from working on anxiety issues using psychological support, from relaxation techniques and yoga to cognitive behavior therapy and hypnotherapy (clinical hypnosis). Both hypnotherapy and cognitive behavior therapy lead to changes in the physiology of the gut and presumably work by helping both anxiety and the production of gut symptoms. More information and a list of health professionals providing hypnosis treatment for IBS can be found at www.ibshypnosis.com.

It may be that other food components are the triggers for your IBS symptoms. Some people have tried wider carbohydrate restriction through elimination of resistant starch and fiber as well as the FODMAPs and reducing the intake of foods containing bioactive chemicals, such as salicylates, amines, and glutamates. If you are considering taking such approaches, we recommend you do so only under the supervision of a registered dietitian; otherwise, you may not get all the nutrients you need.

Another approach is to abandon the FODMAP restriction and undertake an elimination diet, followed by a food rechallenge process. This method is time-consuming and tedious. It should be attempted only under the supervision of an allergy doctor and/or registered dietitian. While skin, blood, and other tests may help identify food hypersensitivities, their interpretation requires the expertise of an allergy doctor.

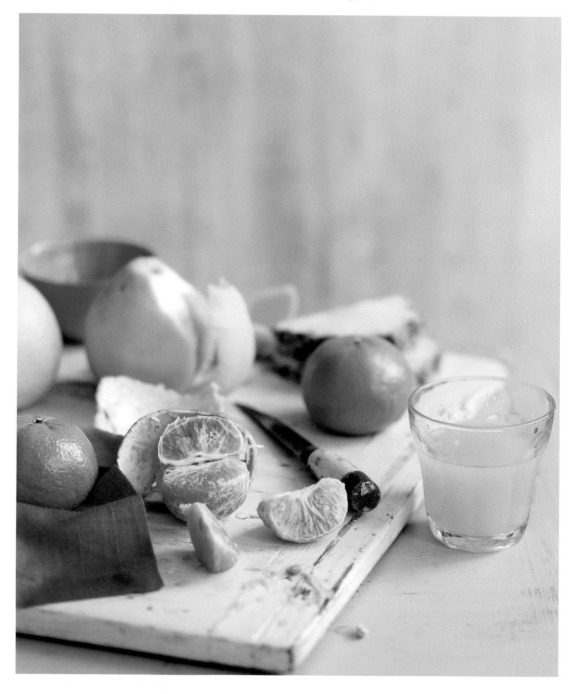

Putting the Low-FODMAP Diet into Practice

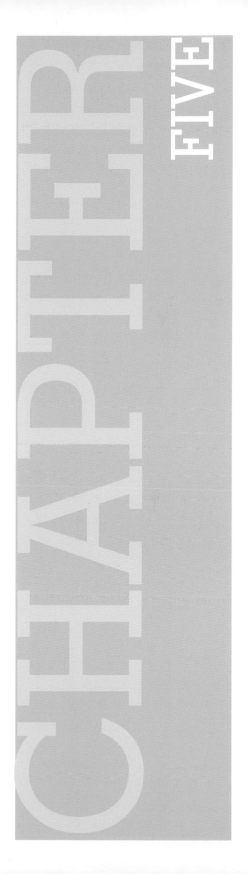

This chapter will help you manage the low-FODMAP diet, whether in an average day at work or home or on a social occasion. There is information on snacks, drinks, how to adapt recipes (although there are plenty of delicious low-FODMAP recipes in this book!), baking hints, and tips for vegetarians, vegans, people with diabetes or inflammatory bowel disease, and children. For easy menu plans, see the next chapter (page 63). And for tips on equipping your kitchen, grocery shopping, and flavoring food, see Chapter 7 (page 78).

Snacks

It would be a waste of hard work if you followed the low-FODMAP diet conscientiously at mealtimes but then ate unsuitable high-FODMAP snacks in between. Here are some great low-FODMAP snack ideas:

- *Fruit*—Fresh fruit makes an excellent snack. See the table on page 45 for suitable fruits, and limit yourself to one piece or a small handful at a time.
- *Vegetables*—Munch on vegetables such as carrots, bell pepper, cucumber, or cherry tomatoes (see page 45 for more).
- *Crackers*—Try suitable gluten-free crispbreads, rice cakes, rice crackers (no onion powder), or corn thins with one of the toppings or cheeses below.
- *Toppings*—Use peanut butter, red meat, chicken, fish, egg, cheese, grated or sliced vegetables, creamed corn, or a small serving of cottage cheese.
- *Cheese*—Enjoy hard and ripened cheeses (see page 32), cheese sticks, cheese wedges, cheese slices, or mini cheeses.

- *Other "everyday" snacks*—Eat yogurt (lactose-free if necessary), popcorn, small amounts of nut and seed mixes (no pistachios or cashews), or a hard-boiled egg.
- *Homemade "sometimes" treats*—Try the following recipes from this book:
  - ➤ *Cakes*—Basic Chocolate Cake (page 211), Vanilla Cake (page 215), Carrot and Pecan Cake (page 216), Moist Banana Cake (page 220), Sweet Almond Cake (page 223)
  - ➤ *Muffins*—Chia Seed and Spice Muffins (page 193), Pineapple Muffins (page 194).
  - ➤ *Cookies*—Chocolate Chip Cookies (page 201), Macaroons (page 202), Simple Sweet Cookies (page 203)
  - ➤ *Bars*—Lemon-Lime Bars (page 204), Strawberry Bars (page 207)
  - ➤ *Other sweet baked goods*—Breakfast Scones (page 197), Lemon Friands (page 219)
  - ➤ *Savory baked goods*—Two-Pepper Cornbread (page 186), Zucchini and Pumpkin Seed Cornmeal Bread (page 189)
- *Commercial "sometimes" snacks*—Try chocolate, potato chips (no onion powder), candy, or ice cream (lactose-free if necessary).

The "sometimes" foods should remain a small contribution to the diet against the background of a nutritious eating plan.

Nonalcoholic beverages

- *Water*—It's the best drink! Drink water in preference to all other beverages, and without restriction. You may like to squeeze lemon or lime juice into the water for a flavor twist.

- **Soda and other soft drinks**—Although these beverages are sometimes sweetened with sucrose and are suitable for a low-FODMAP diet, when sweetened with high-fructose corn syrup, as they typically are in the United States, they should be avoided. Bear in mind that even if you are able to find sucrose-sweetened soft drinks, drinking large quantities will still contribute a large fructose load to your daily intake. Ideally, you should restrict sucrose-sweetened soft drinks to 1 cup per sitting to limit your fructose load. Diet soft drinks are suitable for the low-FODMAP diet.

- **Dairy-alternative drinks**—They include rice milk, oat milk, and quinoa milk. These can be consumed freely as they are lactose-free and low-FODMAP. Soy milks made from soybean extract (not whole soybeans) are usually well tolerated.

- **Sports drinks**—The sweeteners used in electrolyte drinks vary. If they are sweetened with fructose, they should be avoided. Check the ingredients to determine if they are suitable for you to consume, and be mindful about how much you drink at once.

- **Fruit juices**—If these are made from suitable fruits (e.g., orange, cranberry, pineapple, or tomato), they are suitable for the low-FODMAP diet but should still be consumed only in small amounts, typically ½ cup in one sitting. Any more than this may contribute to an excess fructose load. Many fruit-based drinks may include apple or pear juice, even if this isn't indicated in the name of the product. Always read the ingredients of fruit-based beverages to ensure there are no surprise high-FODMAP ingredients.

- **Vegetable juices**—If these are freshly prepared using suitable vegetables, you can drink them freely on the low-FODMAP diet. Many commercially prepared vegetable juices, however, contain onion and should be avoided. If a vegetable juice is tomato-based, drink only ½ cup.

- **Dandelion tea**—This contains fructans and should, therefore, be avoided or consumed only in limited quantities according to your own degree of tolerance.

- **Chicory-based drinks (coffee substitute)**—These are typically made using inulin from the dried root of chicory plants and are high-FODMAP drinks. You should avoid them, or consume them only in limited quantities according to your own degree of tolerance.

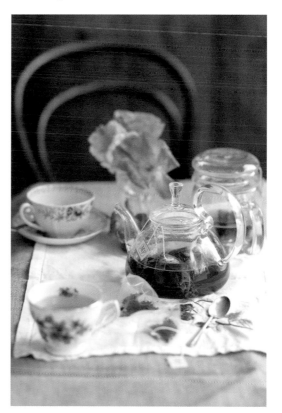

Alcoholic beverages

GENERAL RECOMMENDATIONS

Alcoholic beverages should always be enjoyed only in moderation, but if you have IBS this is even more important, as alcohol in excess can aggravate an irritable bowel. You don't need to avoid alcohol completely, but a sensible, moderate approach will enable you to enjoy a social drink without inducing your IBS symptoms. If you consume alcoholic beverages with food, they are less likely to induce IBS symptoms than if you drink on an empty stomach. This is because the food slows down the release of alcohol from the stomach.

Alcoholic drinks can stimulate your appetite and tend to make you more relaxed. Under these conditions, you may be less likely to adhere to the low-FODMAP diet as strictly as you should. If you wish to consume alcohol, the recommendations are one standard drink for women and two standard drinks for men per day, with two alcohol-free days per week.

ALCOHOLIC BEVERAGES AND THE LOW-FODMAP DIET

The most common potential problem with alcoholic beverages is their fructose load.

- *Wine*—This varies in its sweetness. A standard serving (4 ounces) of dry wine contains minimal sugar and is not a problem, but sweet, sparkling, and dessert wines are high in excess fructose. Examples of dessert wines include fortified wines, such as port, marsala, madeira, muscat, and tokay, and unfortified dessert wines, such as botrytis dessert wines, rice wine, and sauterne.

- *Beer*—Although some types of beer are made from wheat, only a small amount of the wheat remains and is not a problem. Beer, ale, lager, and stout, which all contain gluten, are not suitable for people with celiac disease but are suitable for people on the low-FODMAP diet. As with all alcohol, it is recommended to be consumed in moderation.

- *Spirits*—With the exception of rum, which contains excess fructose, spirits do not contain FODMAPs, even if they are originally derived from wheat or rye. Spirits on their own are suitable for a low-FODMAP diet, but do not consume large quantities because excessive alcohol intake can aggravate the symptoms of IBS. The bigger risk with spirits is usually the mixer.

- *Mixers*—These are usually sugar-sweetened drinks (soft drinks) or juices (such as orange, lime, or cranberry juice). Most mixers have balanced fructose and glucose, but beware of some, such as US soft drinks, which may be sweetened with high-fructose corn syrup. Alternatively, you can use a diet soft drink. Occasionally, milk is used as the mixer, which may be a problem if you have lactose malabsorption. The problem with most mixers lies in the total fructose load if they are consumed in excess. A good rule is to limit your intake to two glasses per sitting.

- *Other alcoholic beverages*—The ones to watch out for are "coolers" and cider. A cooler is a low-alcohol drink made from white or red wine mixed with a soft drink, soda, or juice. Treat them as if they were a fruit juice or soft drink and limit your intake to two glasses per sitting. Cider, an alcoholic beverage typically based on apple or pear juice, is unsuitable for the low-FODMAP diet.

Main meal substitutions

Part Two of this book includes a range of great-tasting low-FODMAP recipes that you, your friends, and the whole family can enjoy (see page 93). You might also like to adapt one of your own favorite recipes so that it is low in FODMAPs. One easy example is changing a quiche recipe to a crustless frittata (like the Sweet Potato, Blue Cheese, and Spinach Frittata on page 131). You can also adapt pizza and pasta dishes by using suitable sauces and gluten-free

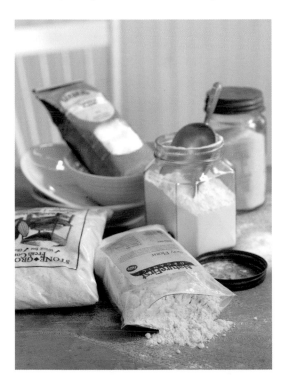

crusts and pasta, which are more and more readily available. If you are not confident that packaged foods are low-FODMAP, cook your meals using basic unprocessed ingredients.

We recommend that if you share meals with other members of your household, you serve everyone the same low-FODMAP dishes. The other members of your household will still be able to enjoy high-FODMAP foods for breakfast and lunch, but you will save time, confusion, and dirty dishes if you don't cook two separate dinners. The low-FODMAP diet is not a bland, tasteless diet at all. If you miss onions, see the tips on page 79 for boosting the flavor of your food.

Basic baking tips

No single flour can be substituted directly for wheat flour. None has the same excellent texture, elasticity, and mouthfeel. A combination of wheat-free flours (usually three or more) works best, since different flours contribute different properties. A good wheat-free flour blend is:

- 2 parts fine rice flour
- 1 part soy flour*
- 1 part either potato flour or cornstarch or tapioca flour

Use the table on page 54 to adapt your baking to your low-FODMAP needs. Baking without wheat flour presents more challenges for the chef, but the tips on the following page should make baking more successful.

---

*This contains GOS and fructans, but in small amounts as part of a recipe does not cause IBS symptoms in most people. Assess your own tolerance.

- Xanthan gum, guar gum, and CMC (carboxymethyl cellulose or cellulose gum) can be used as "gluten substitutes" to help improve the elasticity and crumb structure of baked goods. They can also assist in moisture retention. They are available in health-food stores, and, increasingly, in larger grocery stores. As a general guide, add xanthan gum as follows:
    breads—1 heaping teaspoon
    cakes—1 teaspoon
    cookies—½ teaspoon
    muffins—1 teaspoon
    pastry—1 teaspoon
- Use a variety of flours and sift them together three times to ensure even mixing and aeration (or mix well with a whisk to ensure they are well combined). Sift or whisk any leaveners, such as baking powder and baking soda, and vegetable gums together with the flours.
- Wheat-free baked goods (with the exception of those made using almond or hazelnut flours) tend to dry out more quickly than wheat-based goods, so it's a good idea to cut cakes into slices and freeze the extra portions, or make muffins instead. They will defrost well, but if they seem dry or stale, rejuvenate them in a microwave for 20 to 30 seconds on high.
- Use parchment paper to line your cake pans and cookie sheets, and roll your wheat-free pastry between two sheets of parchment paper.
- Wheat-free baking is often less forgiving, so make sure you follow the recipe to the letter. For the best results, ensure that your oven temperature is accurate and follow the suggested baking times.

SOME SUGGESTED LOW-FODMAP FLOUR MIXES

	FINE RICE FLOUR	CORNSTARCH	POTATO FLOUR	TAPIOCA FLOUR	SOY FLOUR*	NOTES
CAKE 1	2 parts	1 part			1 part	You may substitute potato or tapioca flour for the cornstarch.
CAKE 2	2 parts	1 part	1 part			Increase the quantity of eggs for binding and for protein.
COOKIES	3 parts	2 parts			1 part	Fine rice flour is important for texture.
PASTRY	2 parts	1 part			1 part	Add xanthan gum to improve elasticity and assist in rolling.
SCONES		2 parts		2 parts	1 part	Tapioca flour is important for texture.

*This contains GOS and fructans, but in small amounts as part of a recipe does not cause IBS symptoms in most people. You should assess your own tolerance.

The low-FODMAP diet for vegetarians and vegans

A carefully constructed plant-based diet can be very healthy, but it does require some extra planning. Vegetarians, and particularly vegans, need to be careful about getting enough protein and other nutrients, so should include a wide range of nutritious foods and supplements to provide essential nutrients, some of which, like vitamin B_{12}, occur only in animal foods.

LEGUMES AND SOY PRODUCTS

In a vegetarian or vegan diet, GOS and fructans are often consumed in large quantities as a key source of protein. These may include chickpeas, beans (adzuki, black, butter, cannellini, fava, great northern, kidney, lima, lupini, navy, pinto, and mung), edamame (soybeans), and lentils.

Certain soy foods, including tofu, tempeh, and miso, are low-FODMAP because of how they are processed. In addition, soy milk, yogurt, and cheese are usually well tolerated when made from soybean extract, rather than the whole soybean. We suggest that you include soy products in your diet for their nutritional importance, and monitor your tolerance to them. In other words, you need to determine your own threshold of tolerance. If you *can* tolerate these, you can include soy and other legumes.

If you are an ovo-lacto vegetarian and intolerant to legumes and soy-based foods, you will be able to avoid them without compromising your protein intake by consuming adequate amounts of milk- and egg-based foods.

If you are vegan and intolerant to legumes and soy-based foods, you may find it difficult to meet your daily protein needs. Nuts and seeds, cereal products based on high-protein grains and cereals, and protein-enriched milk alternatives will be your best protein sources. Make a conscious effort to eat them in sufficient quantities (and keep in mind that the recommended average daily protein intake for adults is just 5 to 6½ ounces, according to the American Academy of Dietitians).

TIPS FOR ENSURING AN ADEQUATE PROTEIN INTAKE

- Eat nuts (except pistachios and cashews) and seeds daily, nibbling them as a snack or enjoying nut or seed spreads such as peanut butter and tahini.
- Choose low-FODMAP milk substitutes such as protein-enriched rice, oat, and quinoa milks.
- Choose foods such as pasta, breakfast cereals, and breads made from whole grain, high-protein ingredients such as quinoa and chia.
- If you do not follow a gluten-free diet, try seitan (vital wheat gluten). Because it is made up exclusively of protein, it does not contain any FODMAPs.
- You may be able to tolerate well-rinsed canned lentils or chickpeas (up to ¼ cup) better than dried beans, due to their lower FODMAP content.
- If you cannot tolerate legumes, include the better tolerated soy products such as soy milk made from soybean extract, textured vegetable protein, and tofu.
- If you eat dairy, include milk and yogurt (lactose-free if necessary) and cheese.

- If you eat eggs, eat at least two servings per week.

We recommend that you consult a registered dietitian (see page 39) if you are vegan and wish to follow the low-FODMAP diet. Without professional advice, it will be difficult to ensure an adequate intake of vitamin B_{12} and protein and to maintain your energy levels. There are sample vegetarian and vegan low-FODMAP diet menu plans in the next chapter (see pages 68–71).

The low-FODMAP diet and diabetes

Both IBS and diabetes require eating a specialized diet for good health, and the low-FODMAP diet is ideal for both. Below are some low-FODMAP tips for those with diabetes.

- Eat regular meals and snacks and keep the size of your meals moderate. Try not to overeat.

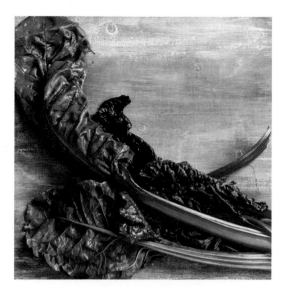

- Eat a variety of foods at each mealtime. Include a carbohydrate source, such as wheat-free bread and cereals, pasta, corn, sweet potato, or rice; a protein source, such as lean red meat, fish, chicken, or eggs; and plenty of appropriate vegetables at each meal.
- Limit high-fat foods, especially those containing saturated fat, such as the skin on chicken, fat on meat, butter, full-fat dairy foods, cheese, cream, coconut milk, take-out foods, and processed meats.
- Avoid trying to balance fructose with glucose to assist with fructose absorption.
- Be cautious about alcohol. Two standard drinks for men and one standard drink for women per day are the recommended maximums for good health. Have at least two alcohol-free days a week, and consider cutting back even further if your food and symptom diary indicates alcohol exacerbates your IBS symptoms.

DIABETES AND THE GLYCEMIC INDEX

A diet for the management of diabetes attempts to control blood glucose levels and maintain a healthy weight. The regularity of meals and the amount eaten are important, as is the choice of foods. To assist with that choice, a ranking system of foods called the glycemic index (GI) has been devised.

The GI ranks foods containing carbohydrates according to how much they raise blood glucose levels. In order to test a food's GI, we monitor a test subject's blood glucose levels every fifteen minutes during a two-hour period after they have eaten a known amount of the food. The higher a food's GI, the faster the blood glucose levels rise, and their peak level will be higher than that caused by a low-GI food. The lower a food's GI, the slower the blood glucose levels rise when it is eaten. This represents a slower but more sustained blood glucose response, which is important for diabetes control.

Although we rarely eat just one food at a time, the lower the GI of each of the food components making up the meal, the lower the meal's total GI will tend to be—similar to the cumulative nature of FODMAPs. Many factors affect GI, including dietary fiber content, the degree to which the grains have been processed, the molecular structure of the starch, and the presence of fat.

THE GI OF LOW-FODMAP FOODS

Many low-GI foods have too many FODMAPs in them and are, therefore, not suitable for the low-FODMAP diet. This applies particularly to wheat-based whole grain foods such as whole grain breads and pasta. Although wheat-free substitutes can have a higher GI, dairy products and many fresh fruits and vegetables have a low GI. Most of these are suitable for the low-FODMAP diet.

LOW-GI TIPS

- Include one low-GI food with each meal to lower the overall GI of the meal, such as (lactose-free) yogurt, suitable low-FODMAP fruit, chia seeds, quinoa, flaxseed, or rice bran with your breakfast cereal.
- Choose foods that are less processed with lots of low-FODMAP whole grains and fiber.
- Add low-FODMAP seeds and nuts to homemade breads.

- Cook your wheat-free pasta al dente (firm to the bite)—this will lower the GI.
- Eat in moderation. Even if a food has a low GI, eating too much of it will have a significant effect on your blood glucose.
- Try to limit juices and soft drinks: Not only are they not suitable in large amounts for the low-FODMAP diet, but they can also contribute to high blood sugar levels.
- Some low-GI, low-FODMAP foods are high in fat or calories and, therefore, are not suitable regular additions to your diet.

The low-FODMAP diet and celiac disease

An entirely gluten-free diet is the only treatment for people with celiac disease, and it must be strictly followed for life (see page 6 for more on celiac disease). This should help improve not only the condition of the small bowel lining, but also other aspects of health, including gastrointestinal symptoms. Some people may follow the gluten-free diet strictly but still experience ongoing gastrointestinal symptoms; in this case, IBS may be occurring at the same time as celiac disease.

If this is the case with you, we recommend that you first consult a registered dietitian (see page 39), to confirm that you are not accidentally ingesting any gluten. It can be difficult to know all sources of gluten that may be present in foods. A registered dietitian is trained to know all the hidden sources, and may identify some that could be the cause of your symptoms. If, however, your dietitian concludes that you have been following a strict gluten-free diet, then you are likely to benefit from trying the low-FODMAP diet in

TIPS FOR SLEEPOVERS

- Explain your child's diet to the host family. See how much they wish to contribute, how adaptable they are, and go from there.
- Pack extra snacks in your child's school lunch so that they will have something to munch on straight after school at the host's house.
- Give the host parents guidelines about suitable dinner options. A simple meal of meat and vegetables is acceptable for most families and will suit your child (provided the meat is unprocessed and the vegetables are suitable).
- Check out the type of cereal usually offered by the host family. If it is unsuitable, pack a serving of cereal for your child to take and some lactose-free milk if lactose intolerant.
- As the host parents become more familiar with your child's needs, you may need to prepare less each time, and you may be able to buy packages of your child's breakfast cereal and bread for the host to keep on hand.

LUNCH-BOX SUGGESTIONS

- Cold roasted red meats, chicken, or hard-boiled eggs with salad
- Wheat-free sandwiches, or bread alternatives, such as rice cakes, gluten-free crispbreads, or corn tortillas, filled with peanut butter (if permitted) or cold meat and cheese
- Vegetable sticks and/or plain corn chips and dip
- Yogurt or a small serving of cottage cheese (lactose-free if necessary)
- A slice of wheat-free pizza
- Quiche (made using wheat-free pastry or a rice crust), a slice of frittata (see page 131), polenta wedges (see page 102), or omelet wraps
- Sushi and sashimi, fried rice (onion-free), rice balls (arancini), or rice-paper rolls
- Fresh low-FODMAP fruit (whole or cut into pieces)
- Plain popcorn or savory muffins
- Leftovers from last night's low-FODMAP dinner

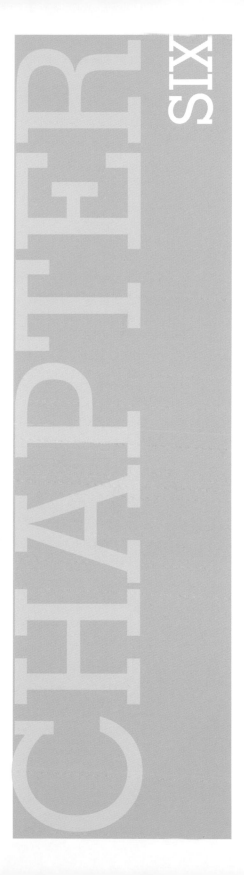

Low-FODMAP
Diet Menu
Plans

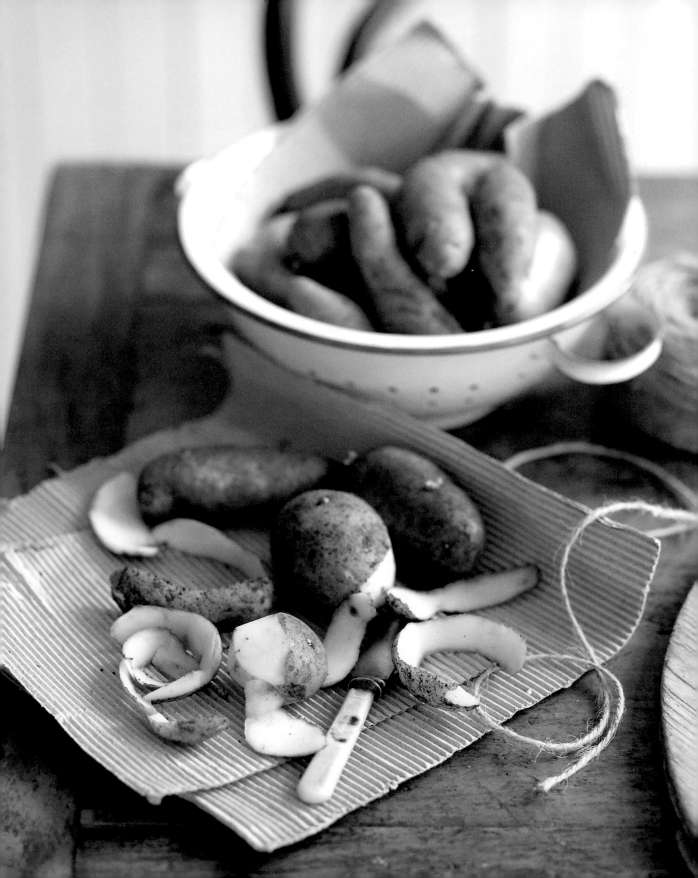

The food plans provided include foods from all food groups and are nutritionally adequate. The low-FODMAP diet can provide you with all the nutrients you need each day, because although some foods are excluded, alternatives are included. The meal plan suggestions are in line with USDA healthy eating guidelines. In general we haven't included quantities, because we all have different energy needs, depending on our gender, age, activity level, and any medical conditions that may impact our health. Unless otherwise unsuitable, we suggest you choose low-fat and low-sodium options whenever possible. A registered dietitian can provide you with individualized dietary advice and your own food plan.

Note that in all the menu plans, LF means lactose-free.

Suitable green vegetables include bok choy, broccoli (½ cup), Brussels sprouts (½ cup), green bell pepper, celery (1 stalk), chayote, Chinese cabbage, fennel (½ cup), green beans, lettuce, peas (⅓ cup), Swiss chard, and spinach.

Suitable orange (or red or yellow) vegetables include red bell pepper, carrots, sweet corn (½ cob), pumpkin or other winter squash, butternut squash (¼ cup), rutabaga, and sweet potatoes (½ cup).

Suitable fruits include bananas, blueberries, cantaloupe, cranberries, durian, grapefruit, grapes, honeydew melon, kiwi, lemons, limes, mandarin oranges, oranges, passion fruit, papaya, raspberries, star fruit, strawberries, tangelos, and tangerines.

GENERAL LOW-FODMAP 14-DAY MENU PLAN

MEAL	DAY 1 MONDAY	DAY 2 TUESDAY	DAY 3 WEDNESDAY
BREAKFAST	gluten-free cereal low-fat milk (LF if required) toasted gluten-free bread butter or margarine jam, peanut butter, or other suitable spread	poached eggs toasted gluten-free bread butter or margarine jam, peanut butter, or other suitable spread	gluten-free cereal low-fat milk (LF if required) toasted gluten-free bread butter or margarine jam, peanut butter, or other suitable spread
LUNCH	Cream of Potato and Parsnip Soup (page 123) gluten-free bread 1 serving suitable fruit	beef sandwich (gluten-free bread, sliced beef, cheese, sliced tomato, lettuce) 1 serving suitable fruit	rice/corn thins or gluten-free crackers with ham, cheese, lettuce, tomato 1 serving suitable fruit
DINNER	Feta, Spinach, and Pine Nut Crêpes (page 138) a suitable green vegetable an orange vegetable ice cream (LF if required) 1 serving suitable fruit	Chinese Chicken on Fried Wild Rice (page 151) sautéed bok choy, celery, carrot, zucchini ice cream (LF if required) 1 serving suitable fruit	Herbed Beef Meatballs with Creamy Mashed Potatoes (page 180) salad (sliced tomato, cucumber, lettuce, celery, bell pepper, olives)

DAY 4 THURSDAY	DAY 5 FRIDAY	DAY 6 SATURDAY	DAY 7 SUNDAY
fruit smoothie (bananas or strawberries, yogurt, low-fat milk [LF if required])	gluten-free cereal low-fat milk (LF if required) toasted gluten-free bread butter or margarine jam, peanut butter, or other suitable spread	gluten-free cereal low-fat milk (LF if required) toasted gluten-free bread butter or margarine jam, peanut butter, or other suitable spread	lean bacon omelet with spinach and tomato toasted gluten-free bread butter or margarine
Cheese-and-Herb Polenta Wedges (page 102) 1 serving suitable fruit	Sweet Potato, Blue Cheese, and Spinach Frittata (page 131) 1 serving suitable fruit	toasted ham and cheese sandwich (gluten-free bread, ham, cheese) salad (tomato, lettuce, bell pepper) 1 serving suitable fruit	Olive and Eggplant Focaccia (page 190) yogurt (LF if required) 1 serving suitable fruit
Peppered Lamb with Rosemary Cottage Potatoes (page 179) gravy a suitable green vegetable an orange vegetable ice cream (LF if required)	Balsamic Sesame Swordfish (page 167) white rice Roasted Vegetable Salad (page 113) Banana Sundaes with Orange Rum Sauce (page 242)	Singapore Noodles (page 152) 1 cup fruit salad (suitable fruits)	Roast Pork with Almond Stuffing (page 176) gravy roasted potatoes, sweet potatoes a suitable green vegetable New York Cheesecake (page 224)

MEAL	DAY 8 MONDAY	DAY 9 TUESDAY	DAY 10 WEDNESDAY
BREAKFAST	gluten-free cereal low-fat milk (LF if required) toasted gluten-free bread butter or margarine jam, peanut butter, or other suitable spread	poached eggs toasted gluten-free bread butter or margarine jam, peanut butter, or other suitable spread	gluten-free cereal low-fat milk (LF if required) toasted gluten-free bread butter or margarine jam, peanut butter, or other suitable spread
LUNCH	egg salad sandwich (gluten-free bread, mashed hard-boiled egg, sliced tomato, cucumber, lettuce) 1 serving suitable fruit	Tuna, Lemongrass, and Basil Risotto Patties (page 101) salad (bell pepper, baby spinach leaves, celery, chopped herbs) 1 serving suitable fruit	ham and cheese sandwich (gluten-free bread, ham, cheese, lettuce, grated carrot) 1 serving suitable fruit
DINNER	Thai-Inspired Stir-Fry with Tofu and Vermicelli (page 155) Citrus Tart (page 231)	Pork Ragout (page 124) cooked gluten-free pasta	Tomato Chicken Risotto (page 158) salad (sliced tomato, celery, lettuce, bell pepper, cucumber) ice cream (LF if required) ½ serving suitable fruit

DAY 11 THURSDAY	DAY 12 FRIDAY	DAY 13 SATURDAY	DAY 14 SUNDAY
gluten-free cereal low-fat milk (LF if required) toasted gluten-free bread butter or margarine jam, peanut butter, or other suitable spread	omelet with spinach and tomato toasted gluten-free bread butter or margarine jam, peanut butter, or other suitable spread	fruit smoothie (bananas or strawberries, yogurt, low-fat milk [LF if required])	poached eggs toasted gluten-free bread butter or margarine jam, peanut butter, or other suitable spread
Lemon Chicken and Rice Soup (page 122) Two-Pepper Cornbread (page 186) 1 serving suitable fruit	Quinoa and Vegetable Salad (page 107) gluten-free bread 1 serving suitable fruit	egg salad sandwich (gluten-free bread, chopped hard-boiled egg, lettuce, mayonnaise) 1 serving suitable fruit	Chicken Noodle and Vegetable Soup (page 121) gluten-free bread 1 serving suitable fruit
Chili Salmon with Cilantro Salad (page 164)	Lamb and Sweet Potato Curry (page 125) cooked rice	Spinach and Pancetta Pasta (page 146) salad (sliced tomato, cucumber, lettuce, bell pepper, celery, olives) Dairy-Free Baked Rhubarb Custards (page 235)	Chicken with Herb Rösti (page 171) a suitable green vegetable an orange vegetable Panna Cotta with Rosewater Cinnamon Syrup (page 236)

LACTO-OVO VEGETARIAN LOW-FODMAP 7-DAY MENU PLAN

MEAL	DAY 1 MONDAY	DAY 2 TUESDAY	DAY 3 WEDNESDAY
BREAKFAST	gluten-free cereal low-fat milk (LF if required) toasted gluten-free bread butter or margarine jam, peanut butter, or other suitable spread	poached eggs toasted gluten-free bread butter or margarine jam, peanut butter, or other suitable spread	gluten-free cereal low-fat milk (LF if required) toasted gluten-free bread butter or margarine jam, peanut butter, or other suitable spread
LUNCH	rice/corn thins or gluten-free crackers with egg, cheese, tomato, lettuce, mayonnaise 1 serving suitable fruit	cheese sandwich (gluten-free bread, cheese, 2 slices tomato, lettuce) 1 serving suitable fruit	Cream of Potato and Parsnip Soup (page 123) gluten-free bread 1 serving suitable fruit
DINNER	Thai-Inspired Stir-Fry with Tofu and Vermicelli (substitute soy sauce for fish sauce) (page 155) Citrus Tart (page 231)	Sweet Potato, Blue Cheese, and Spinach Frittata (page 131) steamed potato a suitable green vegetable an orange vegetable	Feta, Pumpkin, and Chive Fritters (page 97) french fries salad (sliced tomato, cucumber, lettuce, bell pepper, celery) 1 cup fruit salad (suitable fruits) ice cream (LF if required)

DAY 4 THURSDAY	DAY 5 FRIDAY	DAY 6 SATURDAY	DAY 7 SUNDAY
gluten-free cereal low-fat milk (LF if required) toasted gluten-free bread butter or margarine jam, peanut butter, or other suitable spread	omelet with spinach and tomato toasted gluten-free bread butter or margarine jam, peanut butter, or other suitable spread	fruit smoothie (bananas or strawberries, yogurt, low-fat milk [LF if required])	poached eggs toasted gluten-free bread butter or margarine jam, peanut butter, or other suitable spread
Cheese-and-Herb Polenta Wedges (page 102) salad (sliced tomato, celery, lettuce, bell pepper, cucumber) 1 serving suitable fruit	Roasted Vegetable Salad (page 113) gluten-free bread 1 serving suitable fruit	grilled cheese and tomato sandwich (gluten-free bread, 2 slices tomato, cheese) salad (bell pepper, baby spinach leaves, celery, chopped herbs)	Olive and Eggplant Focaccia (page 190) salad (sliced tomato, celery, lettuce, bell pepper, cucumber) yogurt (LF if required) 1 serving suitable fruit
Tofu, Lemongrass, and Basil Risotto Patties (substitute tofu for tuna and vegetable stock for chicken stock) (page 101) sautéed bok choy, celery, carrot, zucchini Banana Sundaes with Orange Rum Sauce (page 242)	Zucchini and Potato Torte (omit the bacon) (page 132) a suitable green vegetable an orange vegetable	Feta, Spinach, and Pine Nut Crêpes (page 138) a suitable green vegetable an orange vegetable ice cream (LF if required) 1 serving suitable fruit	Pasta with Ricotta and Lemon (page 144) salad (bell pepper, baby spinach leaves, celery, chopped herbs) Baked Caramel Cheesecake (page 227)

VEGAN LOW-FODMAP 7-DAY MENU PLAN

MEAL	DAY 1 MONDAY	DAY 2 TUESDAY	DAY 3 WEDNESDAY
BREAKFAST	gluten-free high-protein cereal (containing quinoa, buckwheat, and/or chia) 1–2 tbsp flaxseeds soy* or rice milk toasted gluten-free bread milk-free margarine tahini, jam, peanut butter, or other suitable spread	gluten-free high-protein cereal (containing quinoa, buckwheat, and/or chia) 1–2 tbsp flaxseeds soy* or rice milk toasted gluten-free bread milk-free margarine tahini, jam, peanut butter, or other suitable spread	fruit smoothie (banana or straw-berries, soy yogurt,* soy* or rice milk, chia seeds) toasted gluten-free bread milk-free margarine tahini, jam, peanut butter, or other suitable spread
LUNCH	corn/rice thins or gluten-free crackers with tahini, pesto, sliced tomato, lettuce 1 serving suitable fruit	almond butter sandwich (gluten-free bread, almond butter, celery, grated carrot)	Cheese-and-Herb Polenta Wedges (use soy cheese) (page 102) 1 serving suitable fruit
DINNER	Thai-Inspired Stir-Fry with Tofu* and Vermicelli (substitute soy sauce for fish sauce) (page 155) Rhubarb and Raspberry Crumble (substitute dairy-free margarine for butter) (page 243)	Tempeh* and Sweet Potato Curry (substitute tempeh for lamb) (page 125) white rice nondairy ice cream	Spiced Tofu* Bites (page 104) rice noodles sautéed bok choy, celery, carrot, zucchini nondairy ice cream 1 cup fruit salad (suitable fruits)

DAY 4 THURSDAY	DAY 5 FRIDAY	DAY 6 SATURDAY	DAY 7 SUNDAY
gluten-free high-protein cereal (containing quinoa, buckwheat, and/or chia)	gluten-free high-protein cereal (containing quinoa, buckwheat, and/or chia)	gluten-free high-protein cereal (containing quinoa, buckwheat, and/or chia)	low-FODMAP vegan "sausages"*
1–2 tbsp flaxseeds	1–2 tbsp flaxseeds	1–2 tbsp flaxseeds	toasted gluten-free bread
soy* or rice milk	soy* or rice milk	soy* or rice milk	milk-free margarine
toasted gluten-free bread	toasted gluten-free bread	toasted gluten-free bread	tahini, jam, peanut butter, or other suitable spread
milk-free margarine	milk-free margarine	milk-free margarine	
tahini, jam, peanut butter, or other suitable spread	tahini, jam, peanut butter, or other suitable spread	tahini, jam, peanut butter, or other suitable spread	
Cream of Potato and Parsnip Soup (use rice milk and soy cheese) (page 123)	Roasted Vegetable Salad (page 113)	toasted tomato sandwich (gluten-free bread, sliced tomato, baby spinach leaves, whole grain mustard)	Olive and Eggplant Focaccia (omit the cheese) (page 190)
gluten-free bread	gluten-free bread		1 handful nuts and seeds
1 serving suitable fruit	1 serving suitable fruit	1 serving suitable fruit	1 serving suitable fruit
Tofu,* Lemongrass, and Basil Risotto Patties (substitute vegetable stock for chicken stock and tofu for tuna; omit egg) (page 101)	Stir-Fried Eggplant with Chili and Cilantro (substitute eggplant for pork) (page 156)	Tofu* Kibbeh (substitute tofu* for ground chicken) (page 175)	Risotto Milanese (use soy cheese*) (page 157)
salad (bell pepper, baby spinach leaves, celery, chopped herbs)	1 handful toasted almonds or walnuts	salad (sliced tomato, bell pepper, celery, cucumber, lettuce)	salad (bell pepper, baby spinach leaves, celery, chopped herbs)
nondairy ice cream	white rice	nondairy ice cream	Caramel Banana Tapioca Puddings (use rice milk) (page 240)
	Banana Sundaes with Orange Rum Sauce (page 242)		

* Soy contains GOS and fructans, however products derived from soy such as tofu and tempeh are low in FODMAPs. Also, soy milk, yogurt, and cheese do not cause IBS symptoms in most people if made from soybean extract. You should assess your own tolerance.

LOW-FAT LOW-FODMAP 7-DAY MENU PLAN

MEAL	DAY 1 MONDAY	DAY 2 TUESDAY	DAY 3 WEDNESDAY
BREAKFAST	gluten-free cereal low-fat milk (LF if required) toasted gluten-free bread butter or margarine jam, peanut butter, or other suitable spread	poached eggs toasted gluten-free bread butter or margarine jam, peanut butter, or other suitable spread	gluten-free cereal low-fat milk (LF if required) toasted gluten-free bread butter or margarine jam, peanut butter, or other suitable spread
LUNCH	rice/corn thins or gluten-free crackers with egg, cheese, tomato, lettuce, mayonnaise 1 serving suitable fruit	cheese sandwich (gluten-free bread, cheese, 2 slices tomato, lettuce) 1 serving suitable fruit	Cream of Potato and Parsnip Soup (page 123) gluten-free bread 1 serving suitable fruit
DINNER	Tuscan Tuna Pasta (page 145) salad (bell pepper, baby spinach leaves, celery, chopped herbs) Caramel Banana Tapioca Puddings (use skim milk) (page 240)	Chinese Chicken on Fried Wild Rice (page 151) steamed bok choy, carrot, zucchini, celery 1 serving suitable fruit	Herbed Beef Meatballs with Creamy Mashed Potatoes (use skim milk and low-fat cheese; omit butter in the mashed potatoes) (page 180) salad (bell pepper, cucumber, carrot, lettuce) low-fat yogurt (LF if required)

DAY 4 THURSDAY	DAY 5 FRIDAY	DAY 6 SATURDAY	DAY 7 SUNDAY
gluten-free cereal low-fat milk (LF if required) toasted gluten-free bread butter or margarine jam, peanut butter, or other suitable spread	omelet with spinach and tomato toasted gluten-free bread butter or margarine jam, peanut butter, or other suitable spread	fruit smoothie (bananas or strawberries, yogurt, low-fat milk [LF if required])	poached eggs toasted gluten-free bread butter or margarine jam, peanut butter, or other suitable spread
Cheese-and-Herb Polenta Wedges (page 102) salad (sliced tomato, celery, lettuce, bell pepper, cucumber) 1 serving suitable fruit	Crab and Arugula Quinoa Salad (page 109) gluten-free bread 1 serving suitable fruit	grilled cheese and tomato sandwich (gluten-free bread, 2 slices tomato, cheese) salad (bell pepper, baby spinach leaves, celery, chopped herbs)	Two-Pepper Cornbread (page 186) salad (sliced tomato, celery, lettuce, bell pepper, cucumber) yogurt (LF if required) 1 serving suitable fruit
Peppered Lamb (without the potatoes) (page 179) suitable gravy mixed roasted vegetables with rosemary 1 serving suitable fruit	Balsamic Sesame Swordfish (page 167) roasted potatoes, sweet potatoes a suitable green vegetable white rice Vanilla Cake (page 215)	Singapore Noodles (page 152) 1 serving suitable fruit	Roast Pork with Almond Stuffing (page 176) suitable gravy Roasted Vegetable Salad (page 113) Crêpes Suzette (use skim milk and low-fat margarine) (page 239)

DAIRY-FREE LOW-FODMAP 7-DAY MENU PLAN

MEAL	DAY 1 MONDAY	DAY 2 TUESDAY	DAY 3 WEDNESDAY
BREAKFAST	gluten-free cereal rice milk toasted gluten-free bread milk-free margarine jam, peanut butter, or other suitable spread	gluten-free cereal rice milk toasted gluten-free bread milk-free margarine jam, peanut butter, or other suitable spread	poached eggs toasted gluten-free bread milk-free margarine jam, peanut butter, or other suitable spread
LUNCH	ham sandwich (gluten-free bread, ham, sliced tomato, cucumber, lettuce) 1 serving suitable fruit	beef sandwich (gluten-free bread, sliced beef, sliced tomato, baby spinach leaves, grated carrot) 1 serving suitable fruit	Lemon Chicken and Rice Soup (page 122) Two-Pepper Cornbread (use plant-based milk) (page 186) 1 serving suitable fruit
DINNER	Tuscan Tuna Pasta (page 145) salad (bell pepper, baby spinach leaves, celery, chopped herbs) Caramel Banana Tapioca Puddings (use rice milk) (page 240)	Chinese Chicken on Fried Wild Rice (page 151) sautéed bok choy, celery, carrot, zucchini nondairy ice cream 1 cup fruit salad (suitable fruits)	Spiced Tofu Bites (page 104) french fries salad (sliced tomato, celery, cucumber, carrot, lettuce) nondairy ice cream

The low-FODMAP diet is already low in lactose, but it is not necessarily dairy-free, because dairy products such as cheese and butter are low-lactose foods. However, many people also follow a dairy-free diet, so we have provided a sample menu plan.

DAY 4 THURSDAY	DAY 5 FRIDAY	DAY 6 SATURDAY	DAY 7 SUNDAY
gluten-free cereal rice milk toasted gluten-free bread milk-free margarine jam, peanut butter, or other suitable spread	fruit smoothie (banana or straw-berries, nondairy milk [LF if required]) toasted gluten-free bread milk-free margarine jam, peanut butter, or other suitable spread	omelet with spinach and tomato toasted gluten-free bread milk-free margarine jam, peanut butter, or other suitable spread	poached eggs toasted gluten-free bread milk-free margarine jam, peanut butter, or other suitable spread
Tuna, Lemongrass, and Basil Risotto Patties (page 101) salad (bell pepper, baby spinach leaves, celery, chopped herbs) 1 serving suitable fruit	Egg and Spinach Salad (page 106) gluten-free bread 1 serving suitable fruit	toasted ham sand-wich (gluten-free bread, ham, 2 slices tomato, baby spinach leaves, grainy mustard) 1 serving suitable fruit	Olive and Eggplant Focaccia (omit cheese) (page 190) 1 serving suitable fruit
Lamb and Sweet Potato Curry (page 125) white rice	Balsamic Sesame Swordfish (page 167) white rice a suitable green vegetable an orange vegetable Macaroons (substitute dairy-free margarine for butter) (page 202)	Singapore Noodles (page 152) Dairy-Free Baked Rhubarb Custards (page 235)	Chicken with Herb Rösti (page 171) a suitable green vegetable an orange vegetable Polenta Cake with Lime and Strawberry Syrup (substitute dairy-free margarine for butter) (page 228)

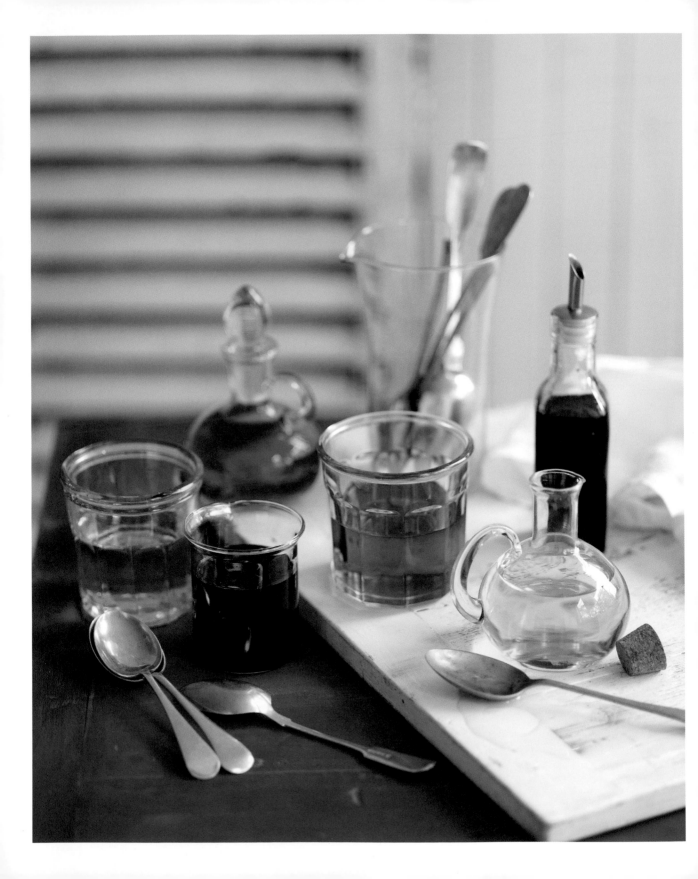

Making the Low-FODMAP Diet Easier

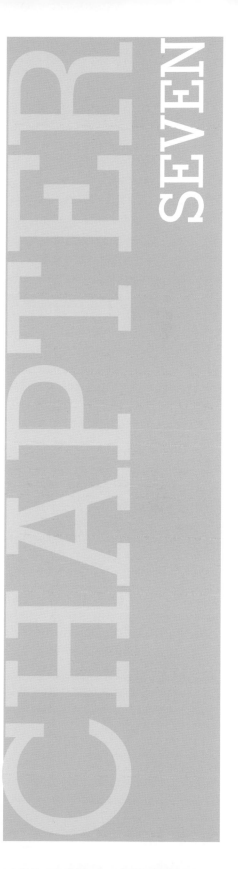

The low-FODMAP diet means changing your cooking methods and what you stock in your pantry. For instance, many people find they miss the flavor of onion in their cooking. But you can boost the flavors of your dishes by using these low-FODMAP herbs and spices: allspice, asafetida, basil, bay leaves, caraway, cardamom, cayenne pepper, celery seeds, chervil, chili, chives, cinnamon, cloves, coriander, cumin, curry, dill, elderflower, fenugreek, galangal, ginger, juniper berries, kaffir lime leaves, lavender, lemon basil, lemongrass, lemon myrtle, lemon thyme, licorice, mace, marjoram, mustard, nutmeg, oregano, paprika, parsley, pepper, peppermint, poppy seeds, rosemary, saffron, sage, sesame seeds, spearmint, star anise, sumac, Szechuan pepper, thyme, and vanilla.

Some people with IBS do not tolerate spicy foods, so use the spices according to your own preferences and tolerance.

Reading food labels

Always read the label to see if a certain food is suitably low in FODMAPs. Ingredients are given in descending order of weight (i.e., the greatest amount is listed first).

As you know, FODMAPs are only a problem when consumed regularly and in significant amounts. If a food contains FODMAP ingredients in more than tiny amounts, you should avoid it. Some foods, however, may contain FODMAP ingredients in too small a quantity to cause gut symptoms, and so can still be eaten. Although honey, for example, is on the FODMAP list, if it is present in very small amounts (such as less than 5 percent of the whole product), then the food would probably be suitable to consume. For more examples, see the table on page 80.

INTERPRETING FOOD LABELS

Here are two examples of how food labels should be interpreted, both with fructose as the FODMAP ingredient.

ORANGE-FLAVORED SPORTS DRINK
The ingredients list reads:

> Distilled water, *fructose,* reconstituted fruit juices (orange, grape), food acid, flavor, preservative

Since fructose is the second ingredient in this sports drink, fructose is present in large amounts and is the main sweetener of the product. We would, therefore, recommend that you avoid consuming this product.

WHEAT-FREE BREAD MIX
The ingredients list reads:

> Corn starch, potato flour, tapioca flour, milk solids, baking soda, salt, fructose, preservative

Since fructose is the seventh (and second-to-last) ingredient in this bread mix, it is present as an incidental ingredient only (less than salt) and does not act as a sweetener in the product. It would be acceptable to consume this product, even though fructose is an ingredient.

Avoiding onion and garlic

The one exception to the rule that small amounts of FODMAP ingredients are suitable to eat is *onion*. We recommend you avoid *all* foods containing onion, even if it is present in minute amounts. Since onion is one of the major triggers of IBS symptoms, it is important to be on the "onion lookout" when purchasing packaged foods such as stocks, gravies, soups, sauces, marinades, potato chips, and other savory snacks such as rice crackers. Onion is not an allergen, so it does not have to be declared on the ingredients list if it is a component of other ingredients. This means that onion could be "hiding" in such ingredients as poultry seasoning, spice blends, vegetable powder, and dehydrated vegetables. These ingredients can also contain hidden garlic, so we recommend that you read the ingredients lists on packaged foods and avoid anything that contains these ingredients, as well as onion, onion powder, and shallots. Note, though, that "natural flavors" or "artificial flavors," when they appear on ingredients lists, will be highly unlikely to cause digestive symptoms, as they are used in very small quantities.

To avoid onion in your meals, look for onion and "hidden" onion ingredients in freshly cooked food and packaged food items, and do not use onion in your own cooking. You should avoid yellow, white, or red onion, shallots, leeks, and the white part of scallions in all your cooking. Alternatives to onion include chives, the green part of scallions (although you should test your own tolerance), fresh and dried herbs and spices, and asafetida, a spice that tastes similar to onion and is available in Indian spice shops.

GARLIC-FLAVORED OIL

Some IBS sufferers can tolerate a small amount of garlic; others cannot. Garlic-flavored oil provides a good flavor substitute. The simplest way to do this when using oil to cook is to place a couple of peeled garlic cloves in the heating oil, brown lightly, then discard the cloves before adding the other ingredients.

There is a wide range of commercially prepared garlic-infused oils available. Because of safety risks, we do not recommend that you infuse your own oil with garlic.

For a quicker alternative, rub your salad bowl with a cut clove of garlic—organic or fresh from the garden is fine—before adding the other ingredients.

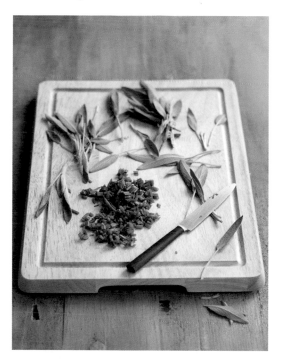

When should wheat be avoided?

Wheat is only a problem ingredient when consumed as a wheat-based carbohydrate food, such as breads, cereals, or pasta (see the list on page 43). Foods that contain minimal amounts of wheat, such as soy sauce or mayonnaise, should not be a problem for people following the low-FODMAP diet.

United States food labeling laws make it compulsory for manufacturers to declare all wheat-derived ingredients, but it is important to realize that many wheat ingredients are actually chains of glucose and do not contain fructans, and so are safe on the low-FODMAP diet. These include wheat starch, wheat thickeners, wheat maltodextrin, wheat dextrin, wheat dextrose, wheat glucose, and wheat color caramel. For those who do not need to avoid gluten, seitan (vital wheat gluten) is also acceptable on the low-FODMAP diet because it does not include the carbohydrates that cause symptoms. For more information on how to read food labels, see page 78.

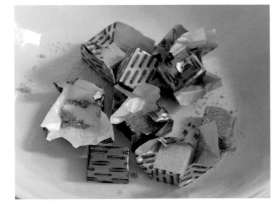

Food additives: what to avoid and what is suitable

HIGH FODMAP: AVOID!	LOW FODMAP: SUITABLE!
isomalt	acidity regulators
maltitol	anti-caking agent
mannitol	antifoaming agent
polydextrose	antioxidants
sorbitol	bulking agents
xylitol	colorings
other ingredients ending in "ol," except for erythritol	color fixatives
	emulsifiers
	enzymes
	firming agents
	flavors
	flavor enhancers
	foaming agents
	gelling agents
	glazing agents
	mineral salts
	preservatives
	propellants
	leaveners
	sequestrants
	stabilizers
	sweeteners (other than those listed to the left)
	thickeners

LOW-FODMAP STAPLES FOR YOUR PANTRY AND FRIDGE

	INGREDIENT*	WHERE TO BUY
FLOURS—ESSENTIAL	cornmeal	supermarkets
	cornstarch	supermarkets
	potato flour	supermarkets, Asian grocery stores, and online
	rice flour (preferably fine rice flour)	supermarkets, Asian grocery stores, and online
	soy flour**	health-food stores and online
	tapioca flour	supermarkets, Asian grocery stores, and online
	arrowroot	supermarkets and online
	buckwheat flour (be aware that some are blends and contain wheat flour)	health-food stores and online
	chickpea flour/besan** (an alternative to soy)	health-food stores, Indian grocery stores, and online
	millet flour	health-food stores and online
	quinoa flour (pronounced "keen-wah")	health-food stores and online
OILS	cooking oil (e.g., canola oil, olive oil, rice bran oil), olive oil spray	supermarkets
SAUCES AND DRESSINGS	fish sauce, hoisin sauce, oyster sauce, soy sauce, garlic-free sweet chili sauce, tomato sauce, mayonnaise, pesto, balsamic vinegar, white vinegar	supermarkets
OTHERS	almond flour, cocoa powder, pine nuts, polenta, vanilla extract, wheat-free bread crumbs, xanthan gum	supermarkets
HERBS AND SPICES	see list on page 78	health-food stores and online

*If following a gluten-free diet, verify that all pantry staples are gluten-free.

**This contains GOS and fructans, but in small amounts as part of a recipe does not cause IBS symptoms in most people. You should assess your own tolerance.

LOW-FODMAP VERSUS GLUTEN-FREE FOODS

A low-FODMAP diet is *not* a gluten-free diet. Gluten-free foods do not contain wheat, rye, barley, or contaminated oats, and so can often be suitable for people on the low-FODMAP diet. People following the low-FODMAP diet can, however, still include oats and usually small amounts of wheat, barley, and rye.

It is important to note that many gluten-free foods contain FODMAPs. Examples include fruits, such as apples and pears, and legumes, such as baked beans.

There are other clear differences between the low-FODMAP diet and gluten-free diets, such as the following:

1. *The diets are treating different underlying problems.* People with celiac disease suffer inflammation in and injury to the small intestine. It is a condition that can lead to serious medical problems if not diagnosed and treated with a strict gluten-free diet for life. IBS, on the other hand, is not associated with injury to the bowel. So, while it causes lots of symptoms and can make life miserable if the low-FODMAP diet is not strictly followed, it does not have potentially serious medical consequences.

2. *One requires absolute restriction and the other only a reduced dose.* People with celiac disease *must* remove absolutely *all* gluten from their diet so that their intestine heals and remains

healed. With the low-FODMAP diet, however, it is all about dose—a small amount of FODMAPs is okay, but larger amounts can cause symptoms.

3. *The consequences of breaking the diet are vastly different.* When someone with celiac disease consumes gluten, they often experience gut and other symptoms, such as "brain fog," and even a flare-up of gut inflammation with a slow recovery. When someone on the low-FODMAP diet consumes large amounts of FODMAPs, they will also experience many symptoms, but these will resolve once the FODMAPs have left the gut, and there will be no ongoing consequences.

4. *One allows flexibility and the other none.* A gluten-free diet is a very strict diet; people with celiac disease who stray from it do significant damage to their bodies. The low-FODMAP diet is not as strict and, once you know your own tolerances, has much room for flexibility.

The low-FODMAP diet is, therefore, very different from the gluten-free diet, and the two should never be confused. Although they have the common element of avoiding grains such as wheat, the low-FODMAP diet restricts the carbohydrate (fructan) content of wheat, whereas the focus of a gluten-free diet is to avoid the protein (gluten) content of wheat completely.

Special Occasions and the Low-FODMAP Diet

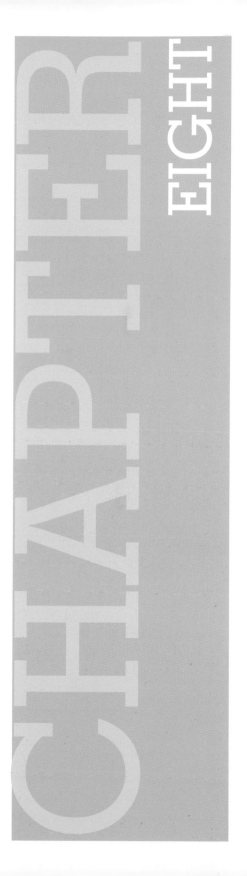

CHAPTER EIGHT

Entertaining at home

MENU IDEAS FOR DINNER PARTIES

Inexpensive
Lemon Chicken and Rice Soup
(page 122)
Zucchini and Potato Torte (page 132)
steamed seasonal vegetables
Caramel Banana Tapioca Puddings
(page 240)

Fancy
Goat's Cheese and Chive Soufflés
(page 137)
Chicken with Herb Rösti (page 171)
steamed baby carrots and wilted spinach
Cinnamon Chili Chocolate Brûlées
(page 246)

Easy
Lemon-Oregano Chicken Drumsticks
(page 169)
Chili Salmon with Cilantro Salad
(page 164)
Rhubarb and Raspberry Crumble
(page 243)

Seafood
Tuna, Lemongrass, and Basil Risotto
Patties (page 101)
Dukkah-Crusted Snapper
(page 166)
Creamy Mashed Potatoes
(page 180)
steamed seasonal green vegetables
Crêpes Suzette (page 239)

Summer
Sweet Potato, Blue Cheese and
Spinach Frittata (page 131)
Balsamic Sesame Swordfish
(page 167)
Mixed Potato Salad with Bacon-and-
Herb Dressing (page 110)
Garden Salad (page 163)
Citrus Tart (page 231)

Asian
Five-Spice Asian Pork Salad (page 114)
Chinese Chicken on Fried Wild Rice
(page 151)
Bananas Sundaes with Orange Rum
Sauce (page 242)

Italian
Olive and Eggplant Focaccia
(page 190)
Spinach and Pancetta Pasta
(page 146)
Frozen Cappuccino (page 249)

Vegetarian
Spiced Tofu Bites (page 104)
Thai-Inspired Stir Fry (omit fish
sauce) (page 155)
jasmine rice
Polenta Cake with Lime and
Strawberry Syrup (page 228)

Dairy-free
Chicken with Maple Mustard Sauce
(page 170)
Roasted Vegetable Salad (page 113)
Dairy-Free Baked Rhubarb Custards
(page 235)

Low-fat

Crab and Arugula Quinoa Salad (page 109)

Prosciutto Chicken with Sage Polenta (page 172)

steamed seasonal vegetables

Sweet Almond Cake (use low-fat yogurt, page 223)

Winter

Cream of Potato and Parsnip Soup (page 123)

Lamb and Sweet Potato Curry (page 125)

jasmine rice

Gooey Chocolate Puddings (page 245)

SUGGESTIONS FOR FINGER FOOD AND PICNICS

Food that is suitable for a cocktail party is often also good for picnics and lunch boxes.

- Feta, Pumpkin, and Chive Fritters (page 97)
- Chicken Tikka Skewers (page 98)
- Tuna, Lemongrass, and Basil Risotto Patties (page 101)
- Cheese-and-Herb Polenta Wedges (page 102)
- Spiced Tofu Bites (page 104)
- Sweet Potato, Blue Cheese, and Spinach Frittata (cut into bite-size pieces for finger food, page 131)
- Zucchini and Potato Torte (cut into bite-size pieces for finger food, page 132)
- Squash, Rice, and Ricotta Slice (cut into bite-size pieces for finger food, page 134)
- Lemon-Oregano Chicken Drumsticks (page 169)

- Breakfast Scones (page 197)
- Lemon-Lime Bars (page 204)
- Lemon Friands (page 219)

For finger food you could also try:

- Strawberry Bars (page 207)
- Mocha Mud Cake (page 212)
- Moist Banana Cake (page 220)
- Sweet Almond Cake (page 223)

And for picnics or lunch boxes you could also try:

- Egg and Spinach Salad (page 106)
- Quinoa and Vegetable Salad (page 107)
- Crab and Arugula Quinoa Salad (page 109)
- Mixed Potato Salad with Bacon-and-Herb Dressing (page 110)
- Roasted Vegetable Salad (page 113)
- Five-Spice Asian Pork Salad (page 114)
- Gluten-Free Fatoush Salad with Chicken (page 117)
- Chicken Salad with Herb Dressing (page 118)
- Chia Seed and Spice Muffins (page 193)
- Pineapple Muffins (page 194)
- Macaroons (page 202)

Eating out

As time passes, you will become very familiar and quite confident in following the low-FODMAP diet at home. You should enjoy the same confidence in restaurants and cafés. Eating at a restaurant should be an enjoyable social experience, so here are some tips for eliminating the stress and cranking up the fun.

If you experience severe symptoms after a small "breakout" from the diet, you'll know to be more strict next time. If, however, you can enjoy a brief deviation from the strict low-FODMAP diet without suffering too many symptoms, then you might choose to be a little less strict when eating out.

LOOK FOR FRIENDLY PLACES TO DINE

If you are new to the low-FODMAP diet, look for establishments that demonstrate an awareness of gluten-free eating and indicate on the menu which options are wheat-free. The waiters in such eateries usually have an understanding of food intolerances and may be more likely to oblige your special requests. Although a low-FODMAP diet is *not* a gluten-free diet, they both restrict wheat. Restaurants and cafés that offer gluten-free options will more likely offer you a more extensive menu. Remember that gluten-free does not necessarily mean low-FODMAP; check that the other ingredients in your meal are also well tolerated.

Some of these establishments offer a dedicated gluten-free menu, others identify gluten-free menu items within the usual menu, and still others state on the menu that they will modify dishes to make them gluten-free. There are various websites available that list "gluten-free friendly" restaurants and cafés.

TELEPHONE AHEAD

If the restaurant or café does not specifically advertise gluten-free or wheat-free meals, it is always a good idea to phone in advance and explain your special dietary needs to the chef. Chefs are becoming increasingly aware of food intolerances. Even if they don't recognize

names like "the low-FODMAP diet," you can still explain your special dietary needs, so that they understand your requirements. Tell them what you can and can't eat. Ask about the ingredients in specific dishes. Give them enough information to help you—without information overload. You could even send a list of foods to the restaurant. This may feel daunting at first, but confidence builds with practice. The chef may be able to advise which meals would be suitable for you or even prepare you a special dish. Reiterate your requirements when you arrive at the restaurant to ensure the meal that arrives is low in FODMAPs.

The following points might help you enjoy a low-FODMAP dining experience, but use them as a guide only. Ask as many questions as you need to feel confident that your meal is low in FODMAPs.

- Write a summary of your low-FODMAP diet on a business-card-size menu card and carry it in your wallet to use when explaining your dietary needs. A registered dietitian could help you with this.
- A "gluten-free meal with no garlic or onion" is a simplified description of the low-FODMAP diet that is easy for waiters and chefs to understand.
- Small amounts of wheat can generally be tolerated by IBS sufferers—you do not need to avoid every crumb on the low-FODMAP diet. This means that you need not religiously avoid bread crumbs on vegetables or a schnitzel, or croutons in salads. If you do wish to avoid even these small amounts of wheat, ask for your meal to be prepared without them, or just leave them on the side of your plate.

- Wheat as an ingredient in sauces (such as soy sauce, teriyaki sauce, malt vinegar, or mayonnaise) is not a problem for the low-FODMAP diet.

- Hidden sources of onion can include stock (used in risottos and soups), gravy, dressings, relishes, and sauces. It may also have been used in marinades for meat and chicken. Sausages often contain onion. Ask for gravies and sauces to be served separately.

- Stuffing in a roast or barbecue chicken contains bread crumbs and usually onion, so it is usually best to avoid the stuffing. Also check the seasoning on top, which could contain onion powder.

- If you break your diet by eating a FODMAP intentionally or unintentionally, you may suffer IBS symptoms, but a break in the diet will not cause any gastrointestinal damage, so you may choose to be more or less vigilant depending on the situation and your anticipated symptoms.

- Some cuisines, such as Japanese, are friendlier than others. The following table lists meals from different cuisines that are often low in FODMAPs, or will require little modification to become so.

LOW-FODMAP SELECTIONS FROM DIFFERENT CUISINES

CUISINE	LIKELY LOW-FODMAP DISHES
Middle Eastern and Indian	kebabs (skewered meat); tikka dishes (yogurt marinade); tandoori dishes; plain cooked rice; kheer (rice pudding—note: contains milk and often pistachios); kulfi (Indian ice cream—note: contains milk and often pistachios)
Southeast Asian	fried rice (check that there is no scallion); steamed or sticky rice; rice paper rolls; sushi (check the fillings); omelets (check the fillings); steamed fish; chili, ginger, or peppered shrimp, meat, fish, or poultry; roast duck or pork; steamed and stir-fried vegetables; rice noodle soup; stir-fries (request no onion or scallion and check the sauces); sweet sticky rice; sorbets (check the flavors)
Italian	risotto (ask for no onion and garlic and check for onion-free stock); gluten-free pasta with pesto (check for garlic), carbonara, or many marinara sauces; steamed mussels; grilled chicken breast or veal steak; shrimp cocktail; mozzarella tomato salad; antipasto (no artichokes); polenta; steamed vegetables; gelato (check the flavors); granita; zabaglione (note: contains lactose)
Mexican	plain corn chips with chili-cheese dip (chili con queso); tacos (beef or chicken with shredded lettuce, cheese, cucumber, and sour cream filling—ask for no salsa); tamales (check that there is no onion or garlic); tostadas (topped fried corn tortillas—choose beef or chicken topping with no onion); fajitas (no onion or garlic, ask for corn tortilla); nachos (no salsa, no refried beans, no guacamole); arroz (rice); arroz con leche (rice pudding—note: contains milk); flan; helados (ice cream, sherbet, or sorbet—check the flavors)
Pub food	plain grilled or roasted meat with vegetables (check the gravy and type of vegetables); grilled fish; risotto (check for onion-free stock and suitable vegetables); salads (check the dressings, ask for no onion or garlic); flourless cakes; sorbets; meringues

TAKE YOUR OWN

You may also like to:

- Take your own suitable dressing or sauce (no onion, garlic, or other high-FODMAP ingredients) and use it on a plain salad or stir-fry.
- Take your own wheat-free bread or roll to a sandwich bar and ask them to fill it with your favorite low-FODMAP fillings.
- Take your wheat-free bread or bread roll to a hamburger restaurant where they can provide an onion-free meat patty and fillings.
- Take your own gluten-free pasta to a restaurant and ask them to top it with a low-FODMAP sauce.
- Take your own pizza base to a restaurant and ask them to top it with onion-free sauces and low-FODMAP ingredients.

Before doing any of the above, you may want to call the restaurant in advance to confirm this is all right.

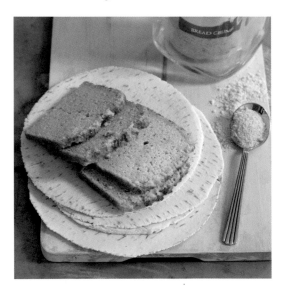

ENJOY YOURSELF!

When your low-FODMAP meal arrives, enjoy it! Relax and appreciate the pleasures of eating out. Afterward, it is kind to provide feedback to the restaurant staff about your dining experience. If you've had a positive experience, you could recommend the venue to your friends and family, and let websites and other restaurant-awareness programs know of your good experience.

Eating at friends' houses

Much of the advice given already is appropriate for friends and family. Why not lend them this book to read, so they can fully understand why you follow a special diet, and what the low-FODMAP diet is all about? Encourage your friends and relatives to read food labels, so they are aware not only of problem foods, but also those that are suitable. If they cook regularly for you, you may wish to provide them with a copy of this book or point them to the book's website, www.thelowfodmapdiet.com. Encourage them to ask questions—the more people understand your dietary needs, the better it will be for you.

It's best not to assume that your friends and family can cater to your low-FODMAP diet. They may forget or make mistakes, not because they don't care, but just because they are only human. To lessen the stress for you and your hosts, here are some useful suggestions:

- ***Ask politely what they intend to serve.*** Then decide if you'd like to ask them to make alterations, or if you would rather self-cater. Discreetly taking your own food will help ensure you don't end up starving all night, and can enjoy food with the others.

- **If necessary, eat before you go**—especially if you know in advance that the menu will not be suitable. You can then just nibble on appropriate snacks during the event. Don't let the food (or lack of it) spoil your good time or anyone else's.

Traveling

Although you have special dietary needs, this should not prevent you from enjoying your travel experiences. The key to a successful vacation is planning, planning, planning!

Airline travel can be difficult, but airline companies are increasingly aware of special dietary needs, and the chances are you will be able to organize a suitable meal. Here are some helpful travel suggestions to ensure you keep your IBS symptoms to a minimum, your taste buds satisfied, and your stomach full:

- Airlines differ in the service they provide— you may need to choose the airline based specifically on the food service it offers.
- Notify the airline of your special dietary need when you book.
- Confirm with your airline a few days before traveling that your special dietary need has been recorded, and check again when you collect your ticket for departure.
- Carry suitable snacks (see examples on page 50) with you just in case there is a problem with your meal.
- You may like to learn some phrases explaining your dietary needs in the languages of the countries in which you'll be traveling.

TIPS FOR TRAVEL WITHIN NORTH AMERICA

Your mode of travel, the time it takes to get there, and the style of accommodation when you arrive are just some of the things you'll need to consider before you leave.

It goes without saying that you are likely to have greater access to specialty foods in larger cities. More remote vacation locations will require a bit more planning on your part, as specialty breads, pasta, crackers, and snack foods will vary in availability. We recommend that you take nonperishable packaged foods, such as breakfast cereal, crackers, and snacks, with you. Safe staple foods such as unprocessed meat, fish, chicken, fruits, vegetables, nuts, seeds, rice, potatoes, milk (though not always lactose-free), and cheese should be available at most destinations.

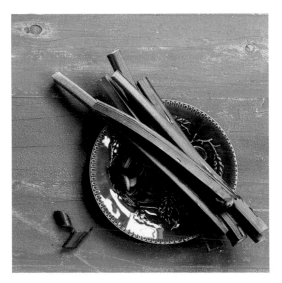

If you have booked a package tour that includes catering, you must organize your special meals *before* you go—it will be quite difficult for the company to arrange a meal for you once you have departed. That way you'll be able to enjoy your dinner and not be restricted to boiled rice, steamed vegetables, and grilled chicken every night.

TIPS FOR OVERSEAS TRAVEL

If you carry specialty foods, such as gluten-free crackers or cereal, with you in your luggage, then you must declare it to customs in most countries. It is advisable to take a letter with you from your doctor stating you have a condition that requires special food. It may also be advisable to contact U.S. Customs and Border Protection regarding food restrictions in other countries.

Awareness of specialty dietary requirements varies around the world. In the United Kingdom, Ireland, Italy, Germany, and Australia, for example, gluten-free products are relatively easy to purchase. In some other European countries, however, especially in Eastern Europe, and across the Middle East, it can be difficult to find wheat-free food products. In many Asian countries, much of the local food is rice-, tapioca-, or potato-based, so it is less challenging to find wheat-free food.

When eating in restaurants overseas, do not assume that the items on the menu are the same as those at home. If possible, find out the ingredients in each item.

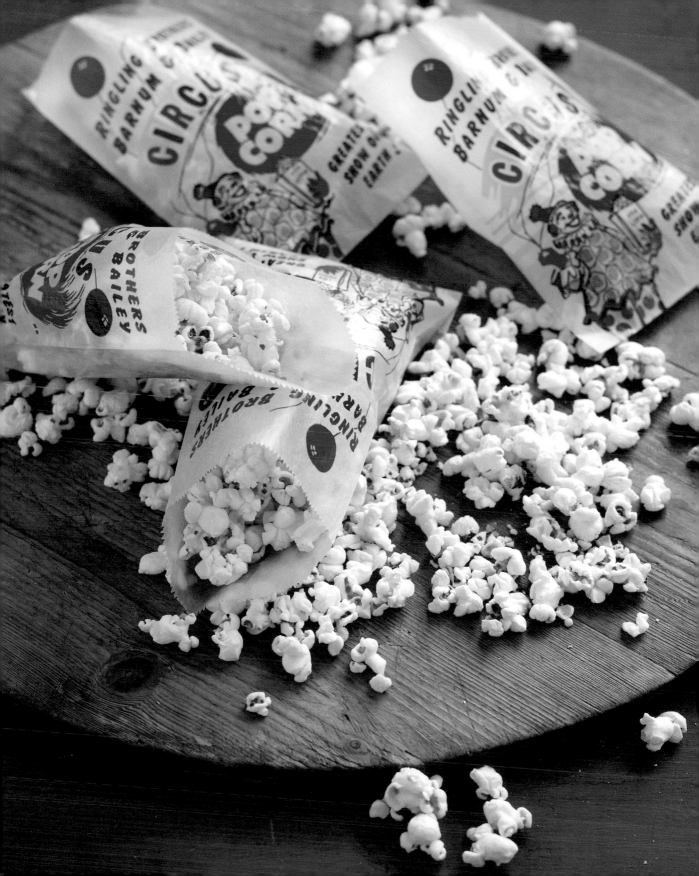

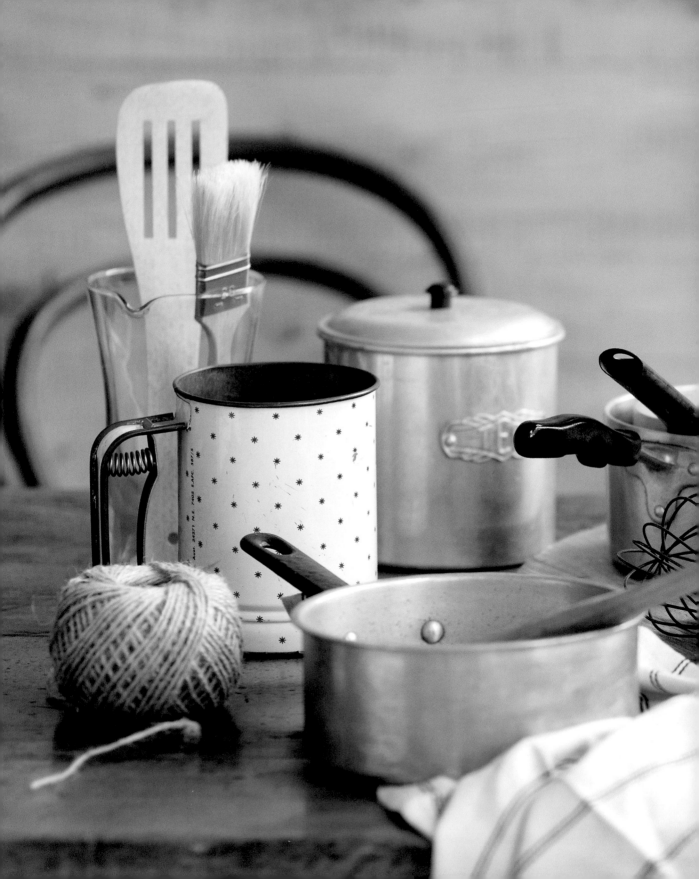

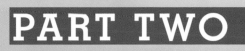

PART TWO

Low-FODMAP Recipes

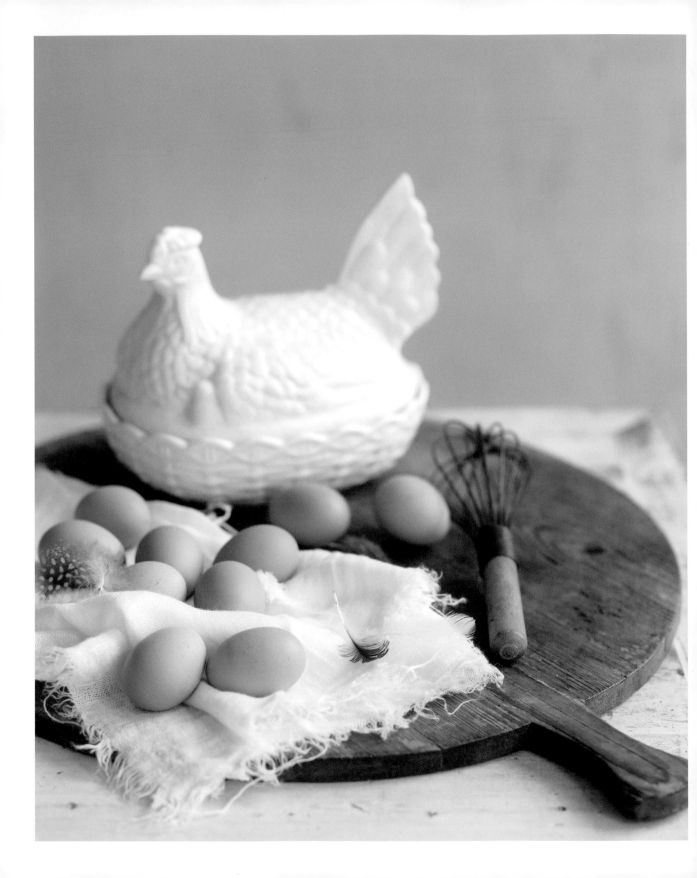

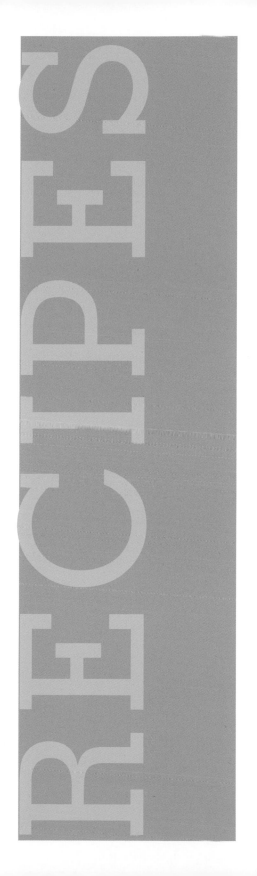

Appetizers and Light Meals

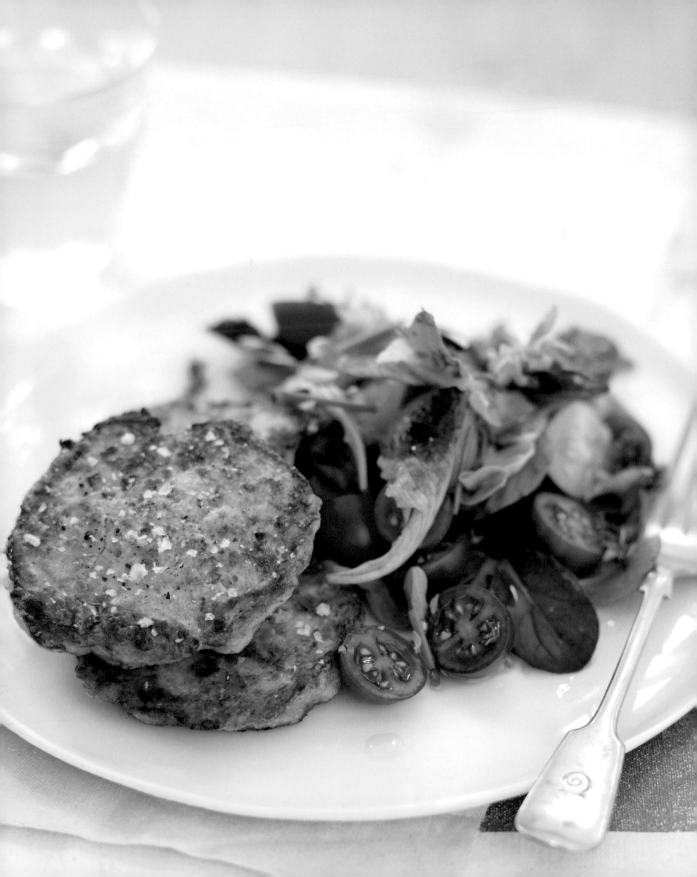

Feta, Pumpkin, and Chive Fritters

SERVES 4

Pumpkin and cumin work so well together, and the addition of salty feta makes these fritters quite irresistible. Eat them just as they are, or serve them with salad and a little sour cream for dipping.

1. Cook the pumpkin in a medium saucepan of boiling water for 8 to 10 minutes, until soft. Drain and mash. Set aside to cool.

2. Sift the rice flour, cornstarch, and xanthan gum into a large mixing bowl (or mix with a whisk to ensure they are well combined). Add 2 tablespoons of the chives, feta, mashed pumpkin, eggs, and cumin, and mix well. Season with salt and pepper.

3. Heat 1 tablespoon of the oil in a medium nonstick skillet over medium heat. Add 2 heaping tablespoons batter per fritter and cook for 2 to 3 minutes. Flip over and flatten slightly with the back of a spatula, then cook for an additional 2 minutes, or until golden brown and cooked through.

4. Transfer the fritters to a plate and cover with foil to keep them warm if eating immediately (otherwise store them in the fridge for later). Repeat with the remaining oil and batter until all the fritters are cooked.

5. Mix together the sour cream and remaining 1 tablespoon of chives. Serve the fritters with salad, if desired, and a dollop of the sour cream topping.

PER SERVING: 294 calories; 9.1 g protein; 15.4 g total fat; 5.2 g saturated fat; 28.2 g carbohydrates; 3.7 g fiber; 200 mg sodium

10 ounces (300 g) pumpkin or other winter squash, cut into ¾-inch (2 cm) pieces (about 2½ cups cubed)

⅓ cup (50 g) fine rice flour

2 tablespoons cornstarch

½ teaspoon xanthan gum

¼ cup (15 g) chopped chives

½ cup (60 g) crumbled feta

2 eggs, lightly beaten

½ to 1 teaspoon ground cumin (to taste)

Salt and freshly ground black pepper

2 tablespoons canola oil

3 tablespoons light sour cream

Garden Salad (page 163), optional

Chicken Tikka Skewers

SERVES 6

If you are using wooden skewers, it is important to soak them in water before adding the chicken—this will prevent them from scorching under the broiler. The marinated chicken is also delicious when threaded onto sturdy toothpicks and served cold or warm as finger food.

1. Combine the yogurt, ginger, garam masala, cumin, coriander, turmeric, and chili in a large bowl, and season with salt and pepper. Add the chicken pieces and stir until they are evenly coated. Cover with plastic wrap and refrigerate for 2 hours.

2. Preheat the broiler. Thread the chicken onto 18 skewers. Place on the broiler pan or a baking sheet and broil, turning to cook on all sides, for 6 to 8 minutes, until golden brown and just cooked through. Serve with salad.

PER SERVING (including 1 cup salad): 335 calories; 45.9 g protein; 13.4 g total fat; 4.7 g saturated fat; 7.1 g carbohydrates; 1.2 g fiber; 100 mg sodium

¾ cup (200 g) Greek yogurt (gluten-free if following a gluten-free diet)

1 tablespoon finely grated ginger

1 tablespoon garam masala

¼ teaspoon ground cumin

¼ teaspoon ground coriander

2 teaspoons turmeric

¼ to ½ teaspoon chili powder (to taste)

Salt and freshly ground black pepper

2½ pounds (1.2 kg) boneless skinless chicken breast, cut into ¾-inch (2 cm) cubes

Garden Salad (page 163)

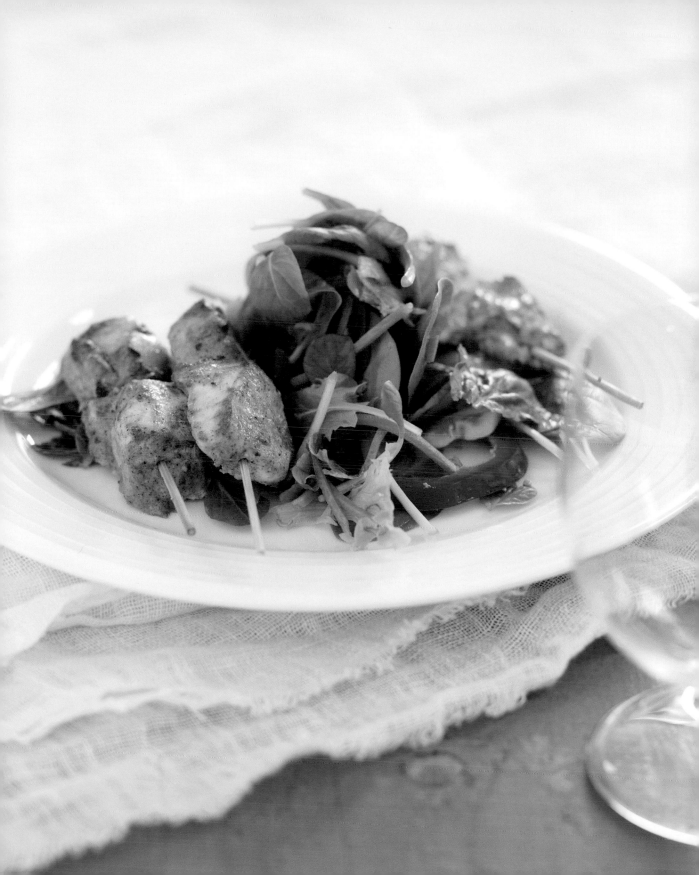

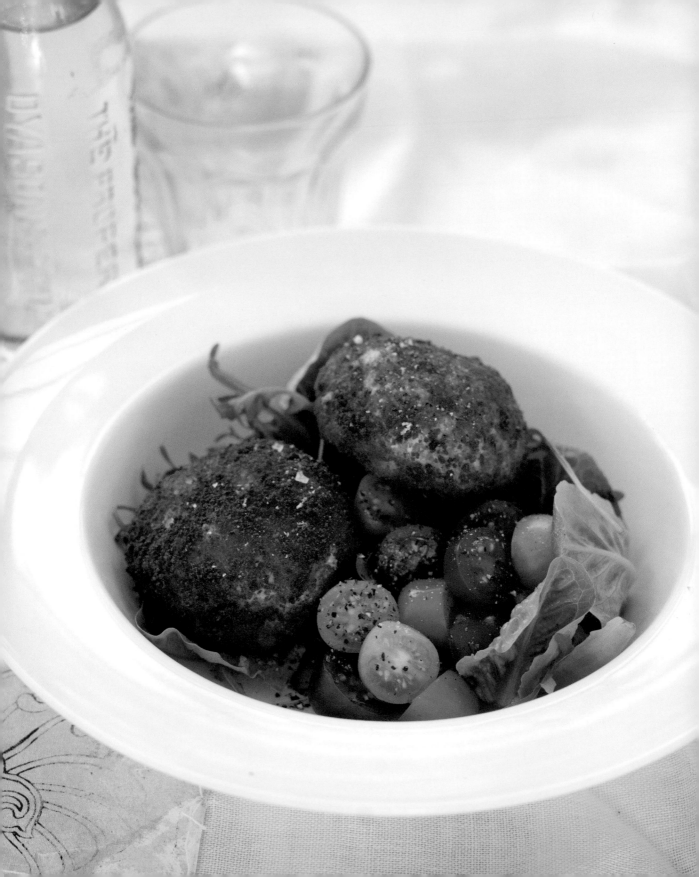

Tuna, Lemongrass, and Basil Risotto Patties

SERVES 4

These flavorful patties are delicious as a main meal with a salad on the side, but they are also great to have as a quick lunch—very transportable and very tasty! For a simple vegetarian option, replace the chicken stock with a suitable vegetable stock, and replace the tuna with 5 ounces of pressed, crumbled tofu (one third to one half of a block).

1. Pour the stock into a large saucepan and bring to a boil. Add the rice and cook for 10 to 12 minutes, until tender. Drain any excess liquid. While still warm, stir in the tuna, lemongrass, and basil, and mix until well combined. Transfer to a medium bowl and set aside to cool to room temperature.

2. Preheat the oven to 300°F (150°C).

3. Stir 1 beaten egg and ⅓ cup (40 g) bread crumbs into the cooled rice, and season with salt and pepper. Form the mixture into 8 large balls, then flatten to make patties. (If the mixture is not quite firm enough, add more bread crumbs.)

4. Place the cornstarch, remaining egg, and remaining 1 cup (120 g) of bread crumbs in three small bowls. Coat the patties with cornstarch, then with the beaten egg, and finally with the bread crumbs. Set aside on a plate.

5. Heat a little oil in a medium skillet over medium-high heat. Add 4 patties to the pan and cook for 2 to 3 minutes, until evenly browned on both sides. Transfer to a baking sheet and keep warm in the oven. Heat a little more oil in the pan and cook the remaining patties. Serve warm with salad.

PER SERVING (including 1 cup salad): 526 calories; 18.2 g protein; 13.9 g total fat; 2.3 g saturated fat; 83.3 g carbohydrates; 1 g fiber; 1,146 mg sodium

3 cups (750 ml) onion-free chicken stock (gluten-free if following a gluten-free diet)

¾ cup (150 g) arborio rice

One 5-ounce (140 g) can oil-packed tuna, drained

2 tablespoons finely chopped lemongrass

2 tablespoons chopped basil

2 eggs, lightly beaten, divided

1⅓ cups (160 g) gluten-free bread crumbs

Salt and freshly ground black pepper

½ cup (75 g) cornstarch

Canola oil

Garden Salad (page 163)

Cheese-and-Herb Polenta Wedges with Watercress Salad

SERVES 4

Polenta is versatile, inexpensive, and satisfying, yet many people have not experienced the pleasure of cooking with it. Here, the polenta is baked until firm, then cut into generous wedges (you could also cut it into smaller pieces to serve as nibbles). Enjoy it hot, cold, or at room temperature.

1. Bring the stock to a boil in a medium saucepan. Pour in the polenta and cook over medium heat for 3 to 5 minutes, stirring constantly—the mixture should be very thick. Stir in the butter, herbs, and ¼ cup (20 g) of the Parmesan.

2. Line an 8-inch (20 cm) square baking dish with parchment paper. Pour the polenta into the dish and smooth the surface. Cool slightly, then refrigerate for 1 hour.

3. Preheat the oven to 350°F (180°C) and line a baking sheet with parchment paper.

4. Turn out the polenta onto a cutting board and cut into 8 wedges or rectangles. Place the wedges on the baking sheet and sprinkle with the remaining Parmesan. Bake for 10 to 15 minutes, until the cheese has melted and the wedges are lightly golden. Alternatively, broil for 5 to 7 minutes.

5. Meanwhile, to make the watercress salad, combine the watercress, cucumber, green and red bell peppers, and alfalfa sprouts in a large bowl. Drizzle with the lemon-infused oil and toss to combine. Serve with the warm polenta wedges.

PER SERVING: 335 calories; 9.7 g protein; 21.4 g total fat; 8.1 g saturated fat; 25.6 g carbohydrates; 3 g fiber; 933 mg sodium

3 cups (750 ml) onion-free vegetable stock (gluten-free if following a gluten-free diet)

1 cup (125 g) cornmeal

2 tablespoons (30 g) butter

⅓ cup (10 g) chopped flat-leaf parsley

⅓ cup (10 g) chopped oregano

⅓ cup (10 g) chopped marjoram

½ cup (40 g) grated Parmesan

WATERCRESS SALAD

4 cups (80 g) watercress

½ small cucumber, halved lengthwise and thinly sliced

½ green bell pepper, cut into ¾-inch (2 cm) strips

½ red bell pepper, cut into ¾-inch (2 cm) strips

3 tablespoons alfalfa sprouts

3 tablespoons lemon-infused olive oil

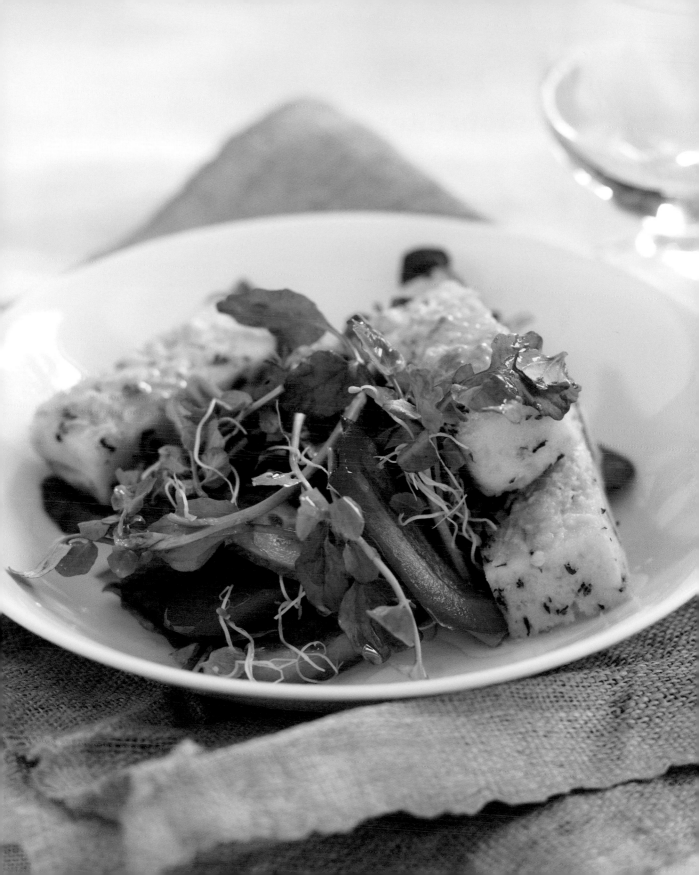

Spiced Tofu Bites

SERVES 4

Tofu is a great vegetarian protein and is tolerated by most people on the low-FODMAP diet. Assess your individual tolerance. This dish uses light, airy tofu puffs, which are available vacuum-packed in the refrigerator section of Asian grocers. If you can't find them, you can substitute pressed, cubed tofu that you have browned briefly in oil.

1. Combine the caraway seeds, pepper, salt, paprika, and allspice in a small bowl, then stir in 2 tablespoons of the oil. Brush the spice mix over the tofu, then transfer to a plate. Cover and refrigerate for 2 to 3 hours to allow the flavors to infuse.

2. Heat the remaining oil in a medium skillet over medium-high heat. Add the tofu and cook for 1 to 2 minutes on each side, until warmed through. Serve with steamed rice and salad.

PER SERVING (including ½ cup cooked rice and 1 cup salad):
489 calories; 13.1 g protein; 30.9 g total fat; 6.8 g saturated fat; 39.6 g carbohydrates; 1.6 g fiber; 288 mg sodium

1 teaspoon ground caraway seeds

½ teaspoon freshly ground black pepper

½ teaspoon salt

¼ teaspoon paprika

¼ teaspoon ground allspice

⅓ cup (80 ml) vegetable oil

14 ounces (400 g) puffed tofu pieces (about 2 x 2 inches/ 5 x 5 cm)

Cooked rice

Garden Salad (page 163)

Salads

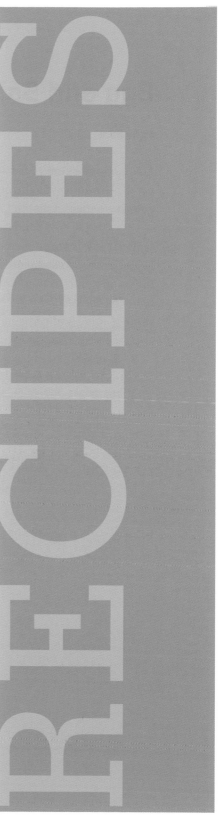

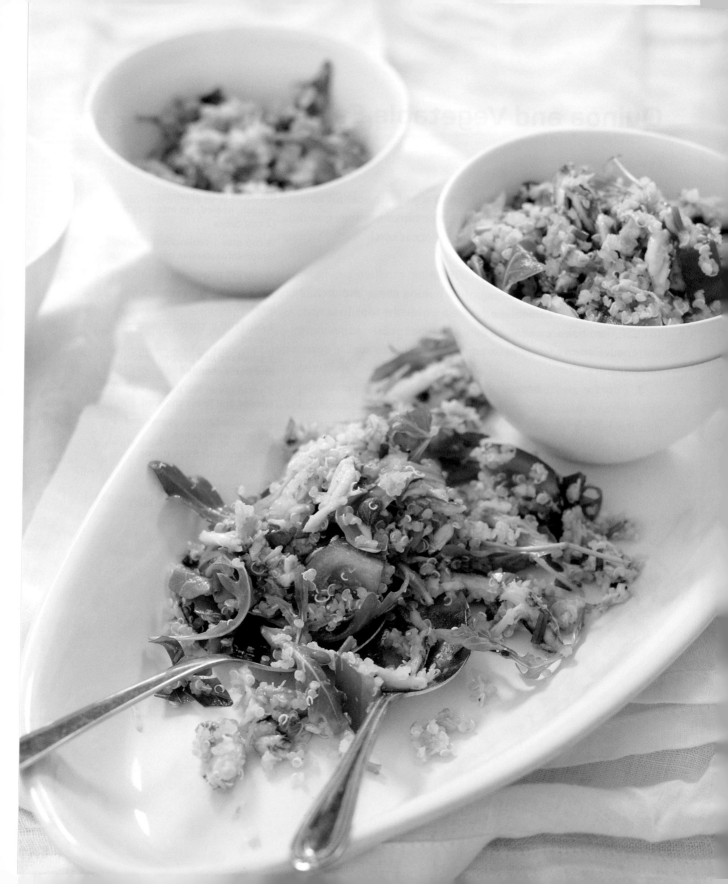

Crab and Arugula Quinoa Salad

SERVES 4

This recipe uses quinoa, an ancient gluten-free grain that is full of nutrients, including a balanced set of amino acids, making it a complete protein source. It has a texture similar to cracked wheat (bulgur)—in fact, in many recipes the two are interchangeable.

1. Pour 2 cups (500 ml) water into a small saucepan and bring to a boil over medium-high heat. Reduce the heat to medium and add the quinoa. Cook, stirring regularly, for 10 to 15 minutes, until all the water has been absorbed and the quinoa is tender. Set aside to cool to room temperature.

2. To make the herb dressing, place all the dressing ingredients in a small screw-top jar and shake well to combine.

3. Combine the quinoa, tomato, crab meat, arugula, and dressing in a large bowl. Cover and refrigerate for 20 to 30 minutes to allow the flavors to meld.

PER SERVING: 313 calories; 24 g protein; 13.1 g total fat; 2.2 g saturated fat; 20.1 g carbohydrates, 8.8 g fiber; 800 mg sodium

½ cup (85 g) quinoa

HERB DRESSING

3 tablespoons extra virgin olive oil

1 tablespoon lemon juice

1 teaspoon grated lemon zest

½ teaspoon finely chopped red chile pepper

1 tablespoon capers, drained

2 tablespoons roughly chopped flat-leaf parsley

2 tablespoons chopped chives

2 tomatoes, chopped

12 ounces (360 g) canned crab meat (two 6-ounce cans)

2 cups (40 g) arugula leaves

Mixed Potato Salad with Bacon-and-Herb Dressing

SERVES 4 TO 6

This is a nice twist on a traditional potato salad, with an added zing provided by the dill pickles and capers. It's sure to be a big hit at your next barbecue.

1. Preheat the oven to 350°F (180°C) and line a baking sheet with parchment paper.

2. Place the sweet potato cubes on the baking sheet, coat with the oil, and bake for 30 minutes, or until tender and golden. Remove from the oven, wrap in foil, and cool to room temperature.

3. Meanwhile, place the red-skin potatoes in a large saucepan and cover with cold water. Bring to a boil and cook for 10 to 12 minutes, until the potatoes are tender when pierced with a fork. Drain, and cool to room temperature.

4. Cook the bacon in a small nonstick skillet over high heat for 3 to 4 minutes, until just crisp, stirring regularly. Remove from the heat.

5. In a small bowl, combine the mayonnaise, sour cream, pickles, herbs, capers, and bacon.

6. Place the cooled potatoes and sweet potatoes in a large bowl. Pour the mayonnaise mixture over the top and gently stir. Season with salt and pepper. Gently stir to just combine, top with the eggs, and serve.

PER SERVING (one sixth of recipe): 365 calories; 17.2 g protein; 18.5 g total fat; 5.2 g saturated fat; 30.6 g carbohydrates; 3.6 g fiber; 1,099 mg sodium

2 small sweet potatoes, washed and cut into ¾- to 1-inch (2 to 3 cm) cubes

1 tablespoon canola oil

6 red-skin potatoes, washed and cut into ¾- to 1-inch (2 to 3 cm) cubes

6 slices bacon, trimmed of fat and chopped

½ cup (125 g) mayonnaise (gluten-free if following a gluten-free diet)

⅓ cup (100 g) light sour cream

¾ cup (120 g) drained and finely chopped dill pickles

1½ tablespoons chopped dill

3 tablespoons chopped flat-leaf parsley

1½ tablespoons capers

Salt and freshly ground black pepper

2 eggs, hard-boiled, peeled, and cut into quarters

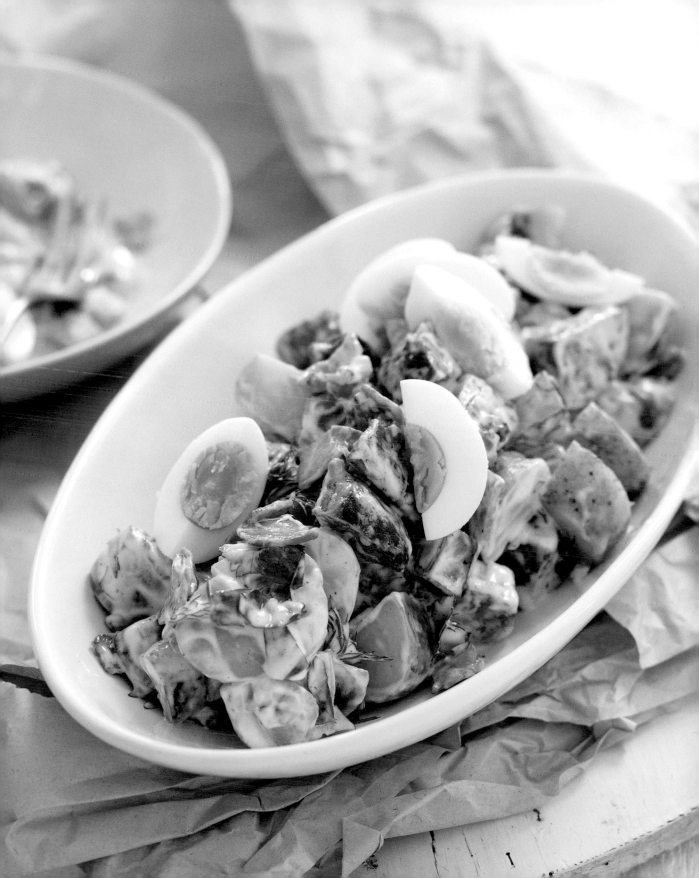

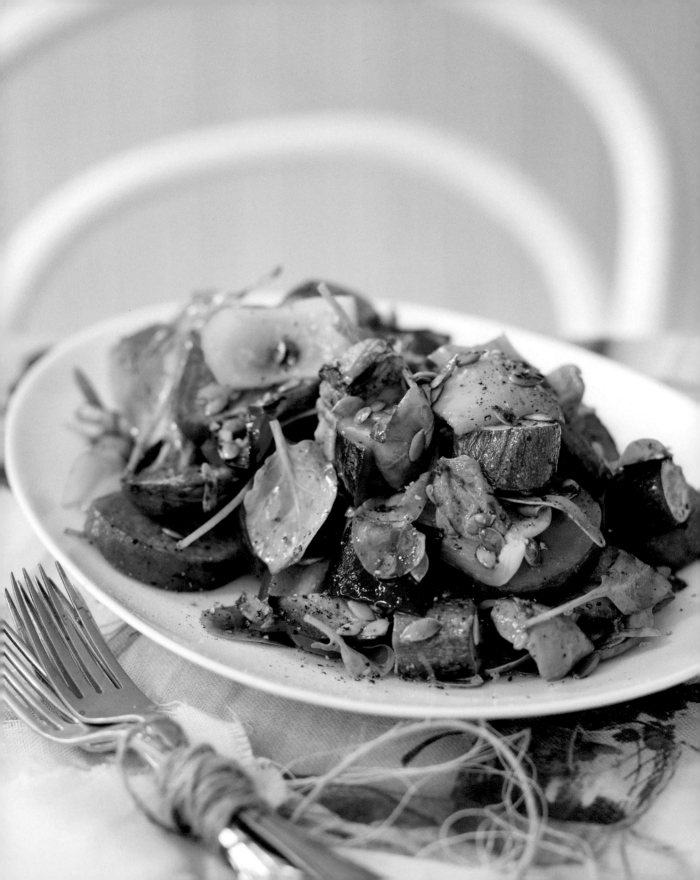

Roasted Vegetable Salad

SERVES 6

This colorful array of roasted vegetables is rich in antioxidants, has a delicious caramelized flavor, and looks great on the plate. With this winning combination, it is sure to become one of your favorite salads.

1. Preheat the oven to 400°F (200°C) and line two baking sheets with parchment paper. Combine the vegetables in a large bowl, drizzle with a little garlic-infused oil, and toss to coat. Place the vegetables on the baking sheets in a single layer and roast for 20 minutes, or until golden, turning occasionally to ensure even browning. Remove from the oven. Cover with foil and cool to room temperature, then place in the refrigerator for 30 minutes.

2. To make the dressing, place the balsamic vinegar and olive oil in a small screw-top jar and shake well to combine.

3. Combine the cooled vegetables and spinach in a large bowl. Add the dressing and toss well, then season to taste with salt and pepper. Top with the roasted pumpkin seeds and serve.

PER SERVING: 317 calories; 15.9 g protein; 18.4 g total fat; 5.2 g saturated fat; 21.2 g carbohydrates; 2.4 g fiber; 1,089 mg sodium

1 eggplant, cut into 1-inch (4 cm) cubes

2 zucchini, cut into thick slices

1 red bell pepper, cut into 1½-inch (4 cm) cubes

1 yellow bell pepper, cut into 1½-inch (4 cm) cubes

2 small sweet potatoes, cut into ½-inch (1 cm) slices

10 ounces (300 g) winter squash, cut into ¾-inch (2 cm) cubes (about 2 cups)

Garlic-infused olive oil

BALSAMIC DRESSING

2 teaspoons balsamic vinegar

3 tablespoons garlic-infused olive oil

3 cups (60 g) baby spinach leaves

Salt and freshly ground black pepper

2 tablespoons roasted pumpkin seeds

Five-Spice Asian Pork Salad

SERVES 4

Ramen noodles are a great crunchy salad topping, but because they are generally made of wheat, they aren't suitable on the low-FODMAP diet. However, if you can locate gluten-free fried rice noodles in the packaged noodle section of your supermarket, they add a great texture to the salad. Otherwise, try sprinkling on crushed peanuts for added crunch.

1. Mix together the canola oil, five-spice powder, fish sauce, vinegar, ginger, and brown sugar in a nonmetallic bowl. Add the pork strips and toss until well coated in the marinade. Cover and refrigerate for about 3 hours.

2. Heat the sesame oil in a wok over medium heat. Add the pork and any leftover marinade, and cook until just cooked through but still tender, 3 to 4 minutes.

3. In a large bowl, combine the lettuce and remaining ingredients with the pork strips and cooking juices. Divide among four bowls and serve immediately.

PER SERVING (including fried rice noodles): 320 calories; 43.5 g protein; 12.8 g total fat; 2.4 g saturated fat; 6.7 g carbohydrates; 2.3 g fiber; 1,241 mg sodium

1 tablespoon garlic-infused canola oil

3 teaspoons Chinese five-spice powder

3 tablespoons fish sauce

3 tablespoons seasoned rice vinegar

2 teaspoons grated ginger

1 tablespoon brown sugar

1 pound (450 g) boneless pork chops, cut into thin strips

2 tablespoons sesame oil

5 cups (150 g) roughly chopped iceberg lettuce

1 cup (50 g) snow pea shoots

½ large cucumber, diced

2 stalks celery, thinly sliced

½ green bell pepper, diced

½ cup (25 g) chopped cilantro or Vietnamese mint

4 ounces (110 g) fried rice noodles, optional

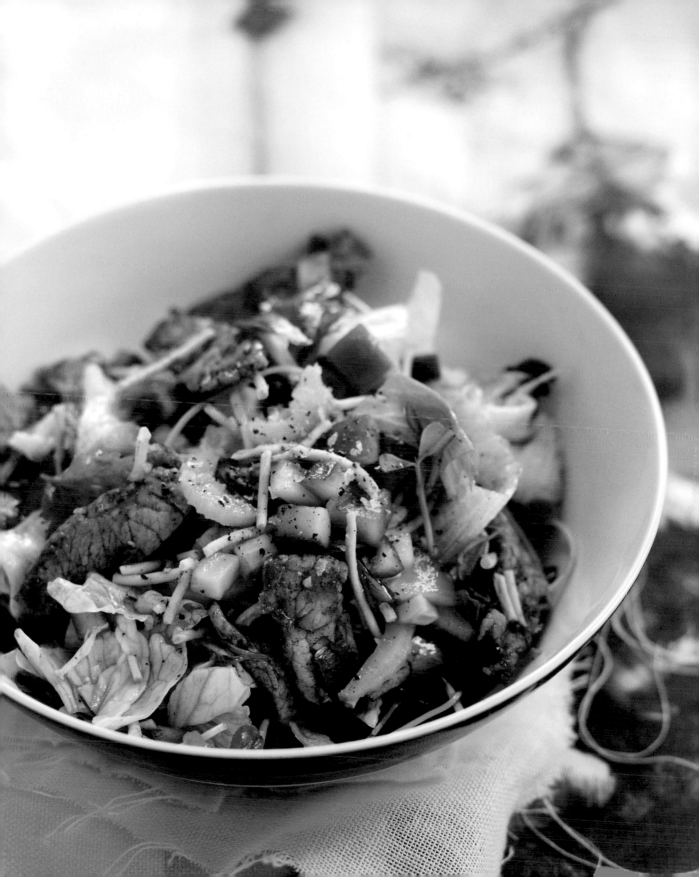

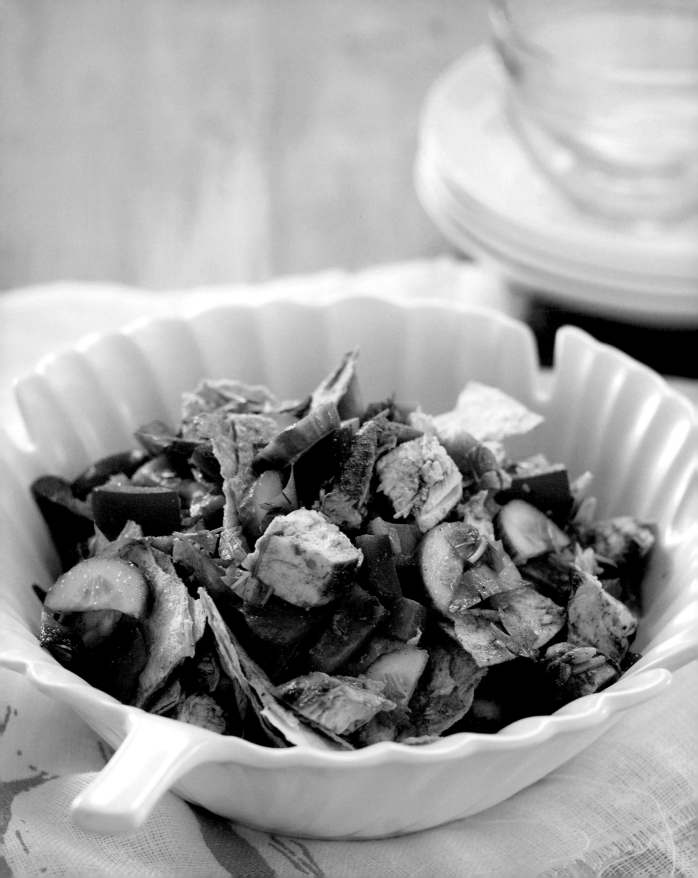

Gluten-Free Fatoush Salad with Chicken

SERVES 4

Gluten-free flatbreads are now readily available in the bread section of larger supermarkets, and may also be found in health-food stores. The main thing with this recipe is to add the toasted flatbread just before serving; otherwise it will go soggy.

1. Mix together the cumin and 1 tablespoon of the canola oil in a small bowl. Brush over all sides of the chicken. Cover with plastic wrap and marinate in the fridge for about 30 minutes.

2. Preheat the oven to 320°F (160°C), or preheat the broiler. Place the flatbreads on a baking sheet and bake for 5 minutes, or just until crisp and lightly golden. If broiling, cook for only 2 to 3 minutes, watching carefully so they do not burn. Once they are cool enough to handle, break into bite-size pieces and set aside.

3. Place the cucumbers, tomatoes, bell peppers, and chopped herbs in a large bowl and toss to combine.

4. To make the dressing, place all the dressing ingredients in a small screw-top jar and shake well to combine.

5. Heat the remaining ½ tablespoon of canola oil in a medium skillet over medium heat. Add the chicken and cook for 3 to 4 minutes on each side, until just cooked through. Remove the chicken from the heat and let it rest for 5 minutes, then cut it into rough cubes.

6. Add the toasted flatbread, chicken, and dressing to the salad, toss gently, and serve immediately.

PER SERVING: 406 calories; 27.4 g protein; 23.9 g total fat; 4.2 g saturated fat; 17.4 g carbohydrates; 2.7 g fiber; 115 mg sodium

1 tablespoon ground cumin

1½ tablespoons canola oil

Two 6-ounce (170 g) boneless skinless chicken breasts

Three 8-inch (20 cm) round gluten-free flatbreads

2 small cucumbers, cut in half lengthwise and sliced

2 tomatoes, chopped

½ red bell pepper, chopped

½ green bell pepper, chopped

½ cup (15 g) chopped flat-leaf parsley

3 tablespoons chopped mint

SPICED LEMON DRESSING

3 tablespoons olive oil

2 tablespoons lemon juice

1 tablespoon garlic-infused canola oil

1 teaspoon ground cinnamon

1 tablespoon ground cumin

1 teaspoon ground cilantro

Salt and freshly ground black pepper

Chicken Salad with Herb Dressing

SERVES 4

We all know that fresh herbs enhance the flavor of a dish, but they are also chock-full of antioxidants. It's a win-win, so I try to add chopped herbs to my recipes as often as possible.

1. Heat 1 tablespoon of the oil in a large skillet over medium heat. Add the chicken breasts and cook for 4 minutes on each side, or until golden brown and cooked through. Remove from the heat and cool to room temperature.

2. Place the mayonnaise, yogurt, cilantro, parsley, and 1 tablespoon of the lemon juice in a small bowl and stir until well combined.

3. Shred the cooled chicken into bite-size pieces and mix into the mayonnaise dressing.

4. Place the lemon zest, remaining 1 tablespoon of oil, and remaining lemon juice in a small screw-top jar and shake well to combine.

5. Place the spinach leaves in a large bowl, add the lemon oil dressing, and toss to coat. Divide the spinach among four bowls and top with the chicken mixture. Sprinkle with toasted sliced almonds just before serving.

2 tablespoons extra virgin olive oil

Four 6-ounce (170 g) boneless skinless chicken breasts

3 tablespoons mayonnaise (gluten-free if following a gluten-free diet)

3 tablespoons plain yogurt (gluten-free if following a gluten-free diet)

1 tablespoon finely chopped cilantro

2 tablespoons chopped flat-leaf parsley

Grated zest and juice of 1 lemon

2 cups (40 g) baby spinach leaves

Toasted sliced almonds

PER SERVING: 360 calories; 46.9 g protein; 17.7 g total fat; 3.4 g saturated fat; 2.9 g carbohydrates; 0.4 g fiber; 153 mg sodium

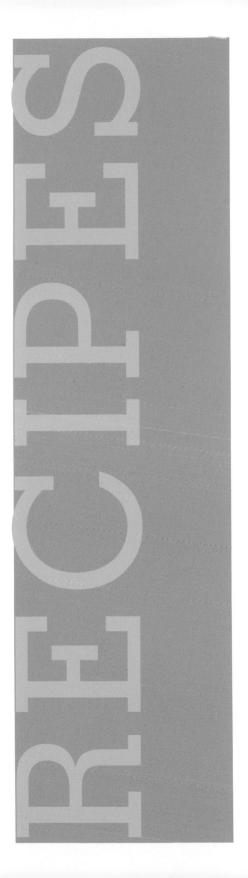

Soups, Stews, and Curries

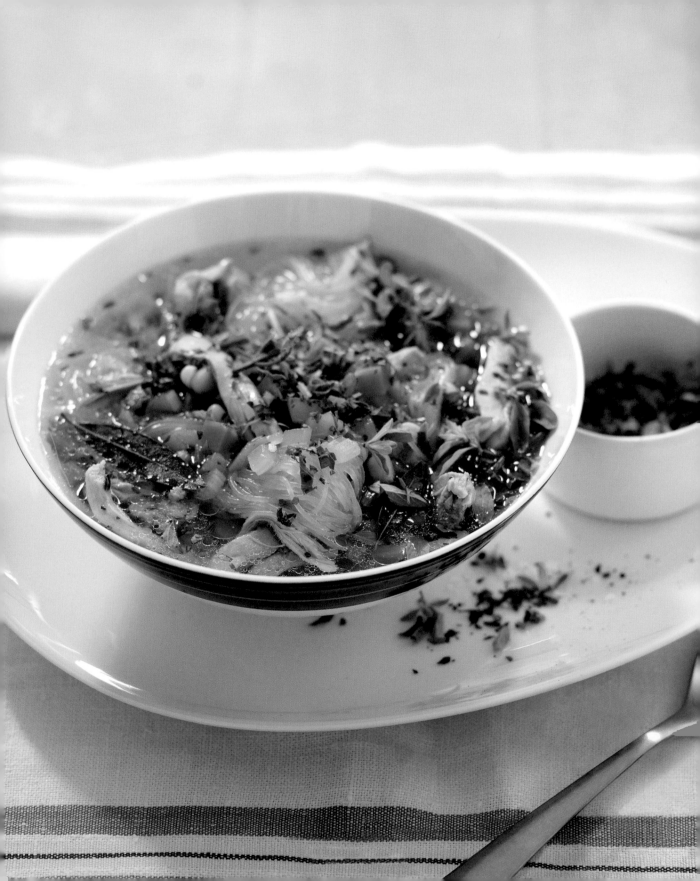

Chicken Noodle and Vegetable Soup

SERVES 4

You can save chicken bones in the freezer or ask a butcher for chicken carcasses. They add a great natural flavor to the soup, so you don't have to rely on bouillon cubes.

1. Heat the oil in a large saucepan over medium-high heat. Add the carrot, celery, bay leaf, and turmeric, and cook, stirring regularly, for 10 minutes, or until the vegetables have softened.

2. Add the chicken carcasses, thyme and marjoram sprigs, and 10 cups (2.5 liters) of water. Bring to a boil, then reduce the heat and simmer, partially covered, for 1 hour. Remove the chicken carcasses and set aside for 10 minutes to cool. Strip the meat from the bones and shred into small pieces. Remove the bay leaf and herb sprigs. Bring the soup to a simmer over medium heat, then add the shredded chicken, sliced chicken thigh, and corn, and cook for 8 minutes.

3. Meanwhile, pour boiling water over the vermicelli noodles and let them soak until they soften. Drain.

4. Add the noodles to the soup and cook for an additional 2 minutes. Stir in the chopped thyme and marjoram, season to taste, and serve with a sprinkling of parsley.

PER SERVING: 316 calories; 22.1 g protein; 14.9 g total fat; 3.1 g saturated fat; 21.3 g carbohydrates; 3.9 g fiber; 233 mg sodium

2 tablespoons canola oil

3 carrots, peeled and finely chopped

2 large stalks celery, finely chopped

1 bay leaf

½ teaspoon turmeric

2 pounds (1 kg) chicken carcasses

5 thyme sprigs, plus 1 tablespoon finely chopped

3 marjoram sprigs, plus 2 teaspoons chopped, or 1 to 2 teaspoons dried

10 ounces (300 g) boneless skinless chicken thighs, thinly sliced

1 cup (175 g) canned corn kernels, drained

1 cup (50 g) rice vermicelli, broken into short lengths

Salt and freshly ground black pepper

2 tablespoons finely chopped flat-leaf parsley

Pork Ragout

SERVES 8

Ragout is the French name for a thick, rich stew that can be made with or without vegetables (this one does feature veggies). It is delicious served with polenta, rice, gluten-free pasta, or mashed potatoes.

1. Heat 2 tablespoons of the oil in a large flameproof casserole or Dutch oven over medium-high heat. Add the pork and cook for 2 to 3 minutes on each side, until browned all over. Remove the pork and set it aside on a plate.

2. Heat the remaining oil in the pot, add the carrot, celery, bay leaves, and sage, and cook, stirring regularly, over medium-high heat for 5 minutes, or until the vegetables soften. Add the stock, tomato puree, potatoes, and pork. Bring to a boil, then cover and reduce the heat to low. Simmer, turning and basting the pork with the liquid occasionally, for 1½ hours, or until the pork is tender. Remove the pork from the pot and let rest on a plate.

3. Increase the heat to medium-high and bring the sauce to a boil. Simmer gently for 20 minutes, or until thickened.

4. Cut the meat from the bone in large pieces and add to the sauce. Season with salt and pepper and serve with polenta, rice, gluten-free pasta, or mashed potatoes.

PER SERVING (including ½ cup of cooked rice): 535 calories; 71 g protein; 10.8 g total fat; 2.2 g saturated fat; 35.8 g carbohydrates; 3.8 g fiber; 496 mg sodium

3 tablespoons garlic-infused canola oil

3- to 4-pound (1.4 to 1.8 kg) bone-in pork leg or center-cut pork loin, trimmed of fat

2 carrots, peeled and diced

2 stalks celery, diced

2 bay leaves

2 tablespoons chopped sage leaves

2 cups (500 ml) onion-free chicken stock (gluten-free if following a gluten-free diet)

One 28-ounce can (825 ml) tomato puree

4 Yukon Gold potatoes, diced

Salt and freshly ground black pepper

Polenta (page 172), rice, gluten-free pasta, or mashed potatoes (page 180)

Lamb and Sweet Potato Curry

SERVES 8

This rich dish achieves its depth of flavor without the use of onion, which is a standard ingredient in most curries. The lamb can be replaced with beef or tempeh if preferred, and any suitable winter squash may be used in place of the sweet potato.

1. Combine the cornstarch, paprika, garam masala, salt, and pepper in a large bowl, add the lamb, and toss to coat.

2. Heat just over half of the oil in a large nonstick skillet over medium heat. Add the curry powder and heat for 1 to 2 minutes, until fragrant. Add the remaining oil, lamb, and celery to the pan, and toss until the lamb is browned on all sides. Stir in the tomato paste, stock, and bay leaf. Increase the heat to high and bring to a boil, stirring often. Reduce the heat to medium-low, add the crushed tomatoes, and simmer for 50 to 60 minutes, until the meat is tender.

3. Meanwhile, cook the sweet potatoes in a small saucepan of boiling water until just tender. Drain.

4. Add the sweet potatoes and spinach to the curry and stir until the spinach has wilted. Serve with rice.

PER SERVING (including ½ cup cooked basmati rice): 507 calories; 36.6 g protein; 22.7 g total fat; 5.6 g saturated fat; 38.0 g carbohydrates; 2.4 g fiber; 566 mg sodium

1 tablespoon cornstarch

½ teaspoon paprika

½ teaspoon garam masala

Salt and freshly ground black pepper

1½ pounds (700 g) boneless lamb loin chops, cut into 1-inch (2.5 cm) cubes

½ cup (125 ml) garlic-infused canola oil

1 to 2 tablespoons curry powder (gluten-free if following a gluten-free diet)

4 stalks celery, sliced

2 teaspoons tomato paste

2 cups (500 ml) onion-free beef stock (gluten-free if following a gluten-free diet)

1 bay leaf

One 14.5-ounce (425 g) can crushed tomatoes

2 sweet potatoes, cut into ½-inch (1 cm) cubes

2 cups (40 g) baby spinach leaves

Cooked basmati rice

Warming Winter Beef Soup

SERVES 6 TO 8

This soup is full of flavor surprises—olives, orange zest, all-spice—but fear not: This unusual combination of ingredients works in perfect harmony to create a very different soup that you are sure to enjoy.

1. Place the cornstarch in a large bowl and season with salt and black pepper. Add the beef and toss to coat.

2. Heat 1 tablespoon of the oil in a large heavy-bottomed saucepan or stockpot over medium-low heat. Add the carrot and celery, and cook for 6 to 8 minutes, until softened and golden. Remove from the pan and set aside on a plate.

3. Heat another 1 tablespoon of oil in the pan and add half of the beef. Cook and toss until browned on all sides, then transfer to the plate with the vegetables. Repeat with the remaining oil and beef.

4. Return the vegetables and beef to the pan. Increase the heat to medium-high and pour in the stock, wine, and tomato puree. Stir well, scraping up any browned bits of meat from the bottom of the pan. Add the orange zest, allspice, and crushed red pepper. Bring to a boil, then reduce the heat to medium-low and simmer for 1 hour, stirring regularly.

5. Stir in the olives and parsley, season to taste, and serve.

PER SERVING (one eighth of recipe): 379 calories; 39.9 g protein; 17.7 g total fat; 4.9 g saturated fat; 10.9 g carbohydrates; 1.7 g fiber; 712 mg sodium

⅓ cup (40 g) cornstarch

Salt and freshly ground black pepper

2 pounds (900 g) chuck beef or beef stew meat, cut into ½-inch (1 cm) cubes

3 tablespoons vegetable oil

2 large carrots, peeled and diced

2 large stalks celery, diced

3 cups (750 ml) onion-free beef stock (gluten-free if following a gluten-free diet)

1 cup (250 ml) dry red wine, or additional onion-free beef stock

1½ cups (420 ml) tomato puree

2 teaspoons finely grated orange zest

¼ teaspoon ground allspice

¼ teaspoon crushed red pepper

1 cup (100 g) pitted kalamata olives, sliced

⅓ cup (10 g) chopped flat-leaf parsley

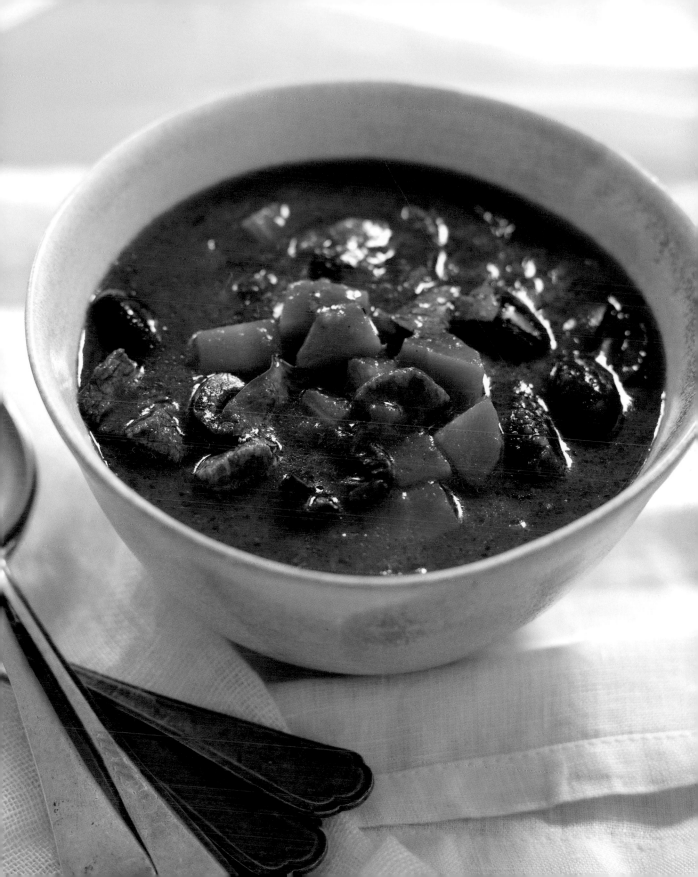

Beef Korma

SERVES 4 TO 6

There is nothing more rewarding than making a flavorsome dish from scratch rather than relying on a prepared sauce. Try this sensational korma curry—you really will be able to tell the difference. If you have lactose intolerance, limit yourself to a half serving only.

1. Heat the oil in a large heavy-bottomed saucepan or stockpot over medium-high heat. Add the almonds, ginger, paprika, coriander, turmeric, cinnamon, cardamom, chili powder, mace (if desired), and cloves, and stir for 30 to 60 seconds, until fragrant. Add the meat and toss to coat with the spices. Cook, stirring, for a few minutes, until browned on all sides.

2. Reduce the heat to low and cook for an additional 5 minutes. Add half of the yogurt and half of the sour cream, then cover and simmer gently for 2 hours, or until the meat is tender, stirring regularly to prevent sticking. Stir in the remaining yogurt and sour cream, and cook until heated through. Garnish with the cilantro and serve with the rice.

PER SERVING (one sixth of recipe, including ½ cup cooked rice):
680 calories; 61.0 g protein; 33.4 g total fat; 11.7 g saturated fat; 33.8 g carbohydrates; 0.8 g fiber; 114 mg sodium

¼ cup (60 ml) garlic-infused canola oil

3 tablespoons ground almonds

2 teaspoons grated ginger

1½ teaspoons paprika

1 teaspoon ground coriander

1 teaspoon turmeric

½ teaspoon ground cinnamon

½ teaspoon ground cardamom

½ teaspoon chili powder

½ teaspoon ground mace, optional

¼ teaspoon ground cloves

2 pounds (1 kg) beef tenderloin, cut into ½-inch (2 cm) cubes

1 cup (280 g) low-fat plain yogurt (gluten-free if following a gluten-free diet)

½ cup (120 g) light sour cream

Cilantro leaves

Cooked rice

Casseroles and Baked Dishes

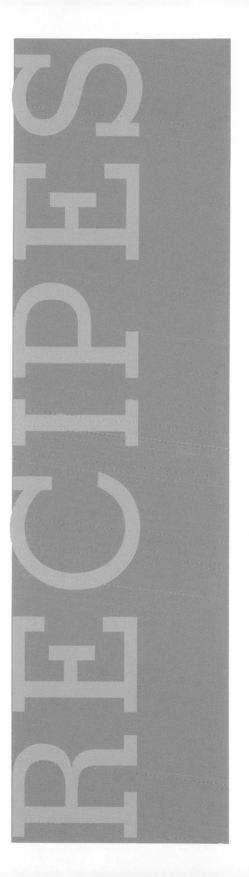

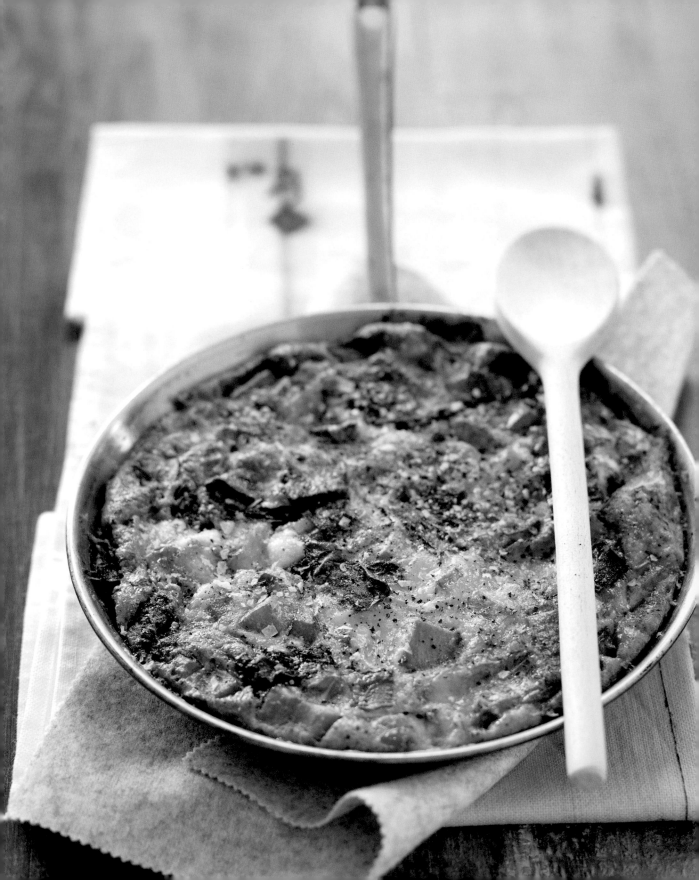

Sweet Potato, Blue Cheese, and Spinach Frittata

SERVES 4

Frittatas are so versatile. You can add whatever ingredients you like to the egg base (although the combination below is totally delicious), then serve them hot, cold, or at room temperature for lunch or dinner, or as finger food. Because blue cheese is considered lactose-free, you can enjoy this dish even if you are lactose intolerant.

1. Preheat the oven to 350°F (180°C).

2. Melt the butter in a 7-inch (18 cm) skillet, preferably one with an ovenproof handle, over medium heat. Add the sweet potato cubes and cook for 10 minutes, or until tender and golden brown. (If you don't have an ovenproof skillet, transfer the sweet potatoes to a greased 9-inch springform pan.)

3. Lightly whisk together the spinach, blue cheese, and eggs in a bowl. Pour over the sweet potatoes, then place the pan in the oven and bake for 20 to 25 minutes, until firm (test by gently shaking the pan).

4. Remove from the oven, then let stand for 5 minutes before slicing. Serve with the salad.

PER SERVING (including 1 cup salad): 368 calories; 22.7 g protein; 24.9 g total fat; 13.2 g saturated fat; 12.7 g carbohydrates; 2.4 g fiber; 579 mg sodium

1½ tablespoons (20 g) butter

2 small sweet potatoes, cut into ½-inch (1 cm) cubes

2 cups (40 g) baby spinach leaves

1 cup (140 g) crumbled strong blue cheese

8 eggs, lightly beaten

Salt and freshly ground black pepper

Garden Salad (page 163)

Zucchini and Potato Torte

SERVES 6 TO 8

This delicious dish can be served hot or cold. Children love it, too, so it is a great one to pack into school lunch boxes.

1. Preheat the oven to 350°F (170°C). Lightly grease an 8-inch (18 cm) square glass or ceramic baking dish.

2. Place the potatoes in a saucepan with 8 cups of lightly salted water. Bring to a boil and cook for 10 to 15 minutes, until tender. Drain. When cool enough to handle, cut into 1/8-inch (3 mm) slices. Layer the potato slices along the bottom of the baking dish.

3. Combine the zucchini, bacon, Cheddar, cornstarch, canola oil, eggs, and salt and pepper in a large bowl. Pour the mixture over the potato slices. Shake the dish to ensure the mixture is evenly distributed over the potatoes. Bake for 45 to 50 minutes, until golden and cooked through. Remove from the oven and let cool for 5 to 10 minutes before slicing and serving.

PER SERVING (one eighth of recipe): 323 calories; 22.8 g protein; 16.7 g total fat; 6.5 g saturated fat; 19.5 g carbohydrates; 2.0 g fiber; 807 mg sodium

3 russet potatoes, peeled

2 large zucchini, grated

8 ounces (225 g) bacon or prosciutto, diced, optional

1½ cups (180 g) grated low-fat Cheddar

½ cup (75 g) cornstarch

2 tablespoons canola oil

6 eggs, lightly beaten

Salt and freshly ground black pepper

Shepherd's Pie

This is a favorite, can't-go-wrong comfort food dinner that is simple to make low FODMAP. Just be sure to choose a suitable brand of gravy powder, and if you add extra vegetables to the mix, be sure they are suitable for you.

1. Preheat the oven to 350°F (180°C). Spray an 8-inch (20 cm) square baking dish with nonstick cooking spray.

2. In a medium saucepan, combine the ground beef, peas and corn, carrot, gravy powder, and water. Cook over medium heat until the ground beef is browned and the gravy has thickened.

3. Meanwhile, cook the potatoes in a pot of boiling water until tender. Drain. Add the margarine and milk, and mash thoroughly, ensuring that there are no lumps and the consistency is very smooth. Add salt and pepper to taste. Add more milk if required.

4. Place the cooked beef mixture into the baking dish. Top with the mashed potatoes. Bake for 20 to 30 minutes, until the mashed potatoes are browned on top.

PER SERVING: 238 calories; 20.4 g protein; 8.5 g total fat; 3.0 g saturated fat; 18.2 g carbohydrates; 2.8 g fiber; 491 mg sodium

1 pound (500 g) lean ground beef

⅓ cup (50 g) frozen peas

⅓ cup (50 g) frozen corn

1 medium (140 g) carrot, grated

¼ cup (40 g) onion-free gravy powder (gluten-free if following a gluten-free diet)

1 cup (250 ml) water

4 large (720 g) potatoes, peeled and quartered

2 tablespoons (30 g) margarine

⅓ cup (85 ml) reduced-fat milk

Salt and freshly ground black pepper

Squash, Rice, and Ricotta Slice

SERVES 4 TO 6

This cooks up into a firm, sliceable rice-based dish, midway between a tart and a casserole. The slice can be enjoyed as a light meal or cut into bite-size pieces to serve as finger food. For those with lactose intolerance, replace the ricotta with feta.

1. Preheat the oven to 350°F (180°C). Grease a 9-inch (22 cm) square ovenproof dish and sprinkle half of the bread crumbs around the base and sides. Invert the dish and shake away any excess crumbs.

2. Bring 2 cups (500 ml) water to a boil in a medium saucepan. Add the rice and cook over medium-high heat for 12 to 15 minutes, until tender. Drain. Return the rice to the pan and stir in the grated squash and zucchini. Cover and set aside.

3. Combine the eggs and cheeses in a large bowl and season with salt and pepper. Add the rice mixture and stir until well combined. Spoon into the prepared dish and sprinkle the remaining bread crumbs over the top. Bake for 45 to 55 minutes, until firm on top when pressed. Remove from the oven and set aside for 5 to 10 minutes before cutting into slices. Serve with salad, if desired.

½ cup (35 g) fresh gluten-free bread crumbs (made from day-old bread)

⅓ cup (65 g) arborio rice

1 cup (200 g) grated winter squash

1 large zucchini, grated

2 eggs, lightly beaten

1¼ cup (225 g) firm fresh ricotta or feta

⅔ cup (50 g) grated Parmesan

Salt and freshly ground black pepper

Garden Salad (page 163), optional

PER SERVING (one sixth of recipe, not including salad): 179 calories; 10.8 g protein; 7.9 g total fat; 4.3 g saturated fat; 16.4 g carbohydrates; 1.7 g fiber; 227 mg sodium

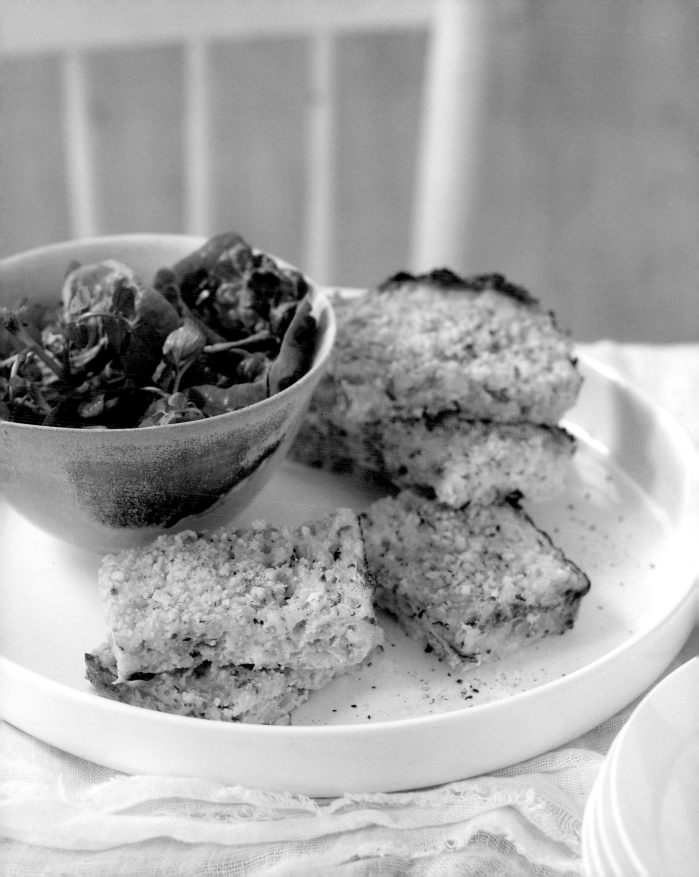

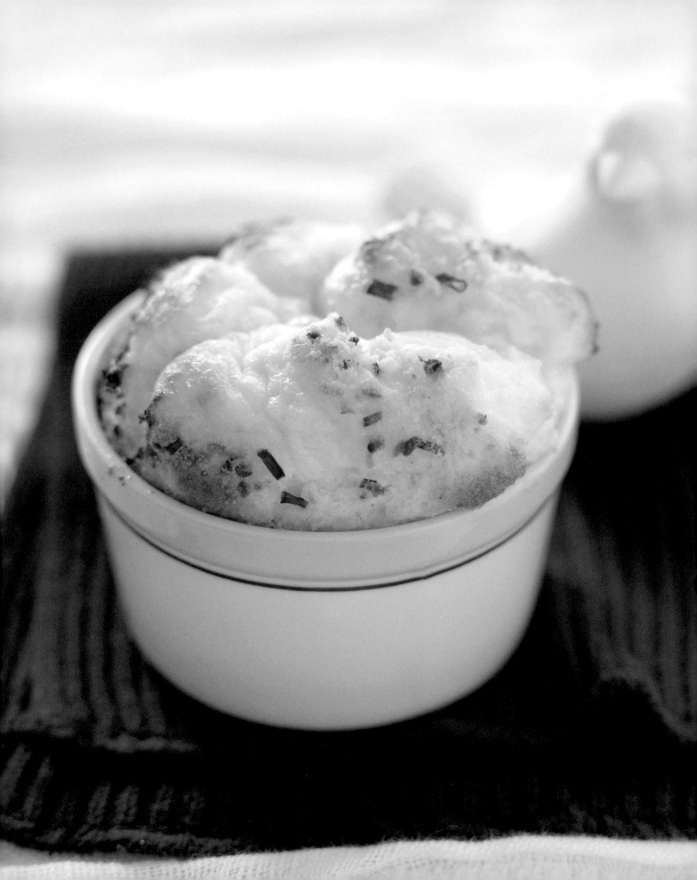

Goat's Cheese and Chive Soufflés

MAKES 6

Baking a soufflé might seem like a daunting task, but it needn't be. I guarantee this dish will be a great success—try it for your next dinner party!

1. Preheat the oven to 350°F (180°C) and line a baking sheet with parchment paper. Grease six 5-ounce (150 ml) soufflé dishes or ramekins and lightly coat with gluten-free bread crumbs. Invert the dishes and shake away any excess crumbs. Place the dishes in a separate shallow baking dish.

2. Melt the margarine in a medium saucepan over low heat. Add the cornstarch and cook, stirring constantly, for 1 to 2 minutes. Slowly pour in the goat's milk and mix to make a smooth paste. Cook, stirring, for an additional 2 to 3 minutes, until thickened.

3. Transfer the mixture to a medium bowl. Add the egg yolks, one at a time, beating well with an electric mixer between additions. Add the goat's cheese, chives, and parsley, and beat until just combined. Season with salt and pepper.

4. Clean the beaters. In a large clean bowl, beat the egg whites until firm peaks form, 5 to 6 minutes. Gently fold into the cheese mixture until well combined. Spoon into the soufflé dishes. Pour enough boiling water into the baking dish to come halfway up the sides of the dishes. Bake for 20 minutes, or until well risen and slightly browned.

5. To make the topping, combine the bread crumbs, chives, and goat's cheese in a small bowl. Season with salt, and mix until evenly fine and crumbly.

6. Remove the soufflés from the oven and place on the prepared baking sheet. Brush with melted margarine and sprinkle with the topping. Bake for 7 to 8 minutes, until puffed with a firm crust. Serve immediately with salad, if desired.

PER SERVING (not including salad): 267 calories; 9.9 g protein; 17.3 g total fat; 7.6 g saturated fat; 18.8 g carbohydrates; 0.1 g fiber; 270 mg sodium

3 tablespoons dried gluten-free bread crumbs

4 tablespoons (60 g) dairy-free margarine

⅓ cup (50 g) cornstarch

1¼ cups (300 ml) goat's milk, lactose-free milk, or suitable plant-based milk

3 large eggs, separated

1 cup (120 g) crumbled goat's cheese

2 teaspoons chopped chives

2 teaspoons finely chopped flat-leaf parsley

Salt and freshly ground black pepper

TOPPING

2 tablespoons fresh gluten-free bread crumbs (made from day-old bread)

1 teaspoon chopped chives

3 tablespoons (20 g) crumbled goat's cheese

Salt

2 teaspoons dairy-free margarine, melted

Garden Salad (page 163), optional

Feta, Spinach, and Pine Nut Crêpes

SERVES 6

Soy flour is quite bitter in its uncooked state, but the bitterness disappears when cooked. The amount of soy flour used in this recipe is minimal, but assess your individual tolerance—if necessary, you can replace the soy flour with tapioca flour.

1. Sift the rice flour, cornstarch, soy flour, and baking soda three times into a bowl (or mix well with a whisk to ensure they are well combined), and make a well in the center. Add the milk and beaten eggs, and blend to form a smooth batter. Stir in the melted butter. Cover with plastic wrap and set aside for 20 minutes.

2. Spray a skillet with cooking spray and set over medium heat. Pour in enough batter to coat the base of the pan when it is tilted, and cook until bubbles appear. Turn and cook the other side. Remove and keep warm. Repeat with the remaining batter to make 12 crêpes in all.

3. Preheat the oven to 350°F (180°C).

4. To make the filling, heat the oil in a large heavy-bottomed skillet over medium-high heat. Add the pine nuts and cook until just browned (watch carefully as they can burn easily). Add the spinach and feta, and stir until well combined. Stir in the egg until just cooked. Season to taste with salt and pepper.

5. Place spoonfuls of the filling across the center of each crêpe and roll up. Place the rolled crêpes, seam-side down, in one large or two small baking dishes in a single layer, and pour the tomato puree evenly over the top. Sprinkle with the Cheddar. Bake for 10 to 15 minutes, until the cheese has melted. Serve with salad, if desired.

PER SERVING (not including salad): 551 calories; 32 g protein; 31.5 g total fat; 15.8 g saturated fat; 33.5 g carbohydrates; 2.5 g fiber; 1,093 mg sodium

¾ cup (100 g) fine rice flour

½ cup (75 g) cornstarch

⅓ cup (30 g) soy flour

¾ teaspoon baking soda

1½ cups (375 ml) low-fat milk, lactose-free milk, or suitable plant-based milk

2 eggs, lightly beaten

3 tablespoons (40 g) butter, melted

FETA, SPINACH, AND PINE NUT FILLING

2 teaspoons canola oil

3 tablespoons pine nuts

One 16-ounce (500 g) package chopped frozen spinach, thawed and squeezed dry

4 cups (500 g) crumbled reduced-fat feta

1 egg, lightly beaten

Salt and freshly ground black pepper

1 cup (280 g) tomato puree

½ cup (60 g) grated low-fat Cheddar

Garden Salad (page 163), optional

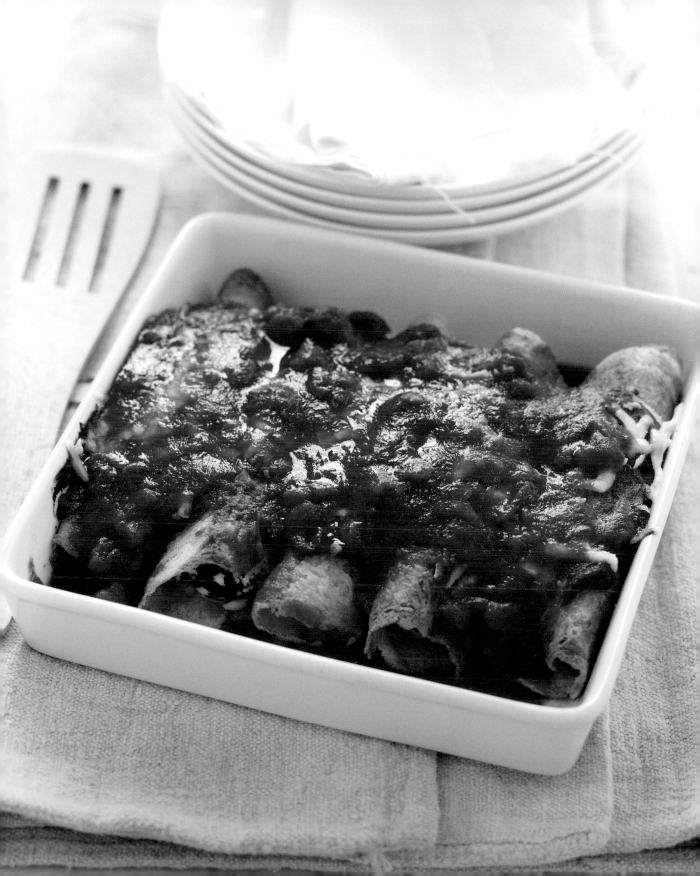

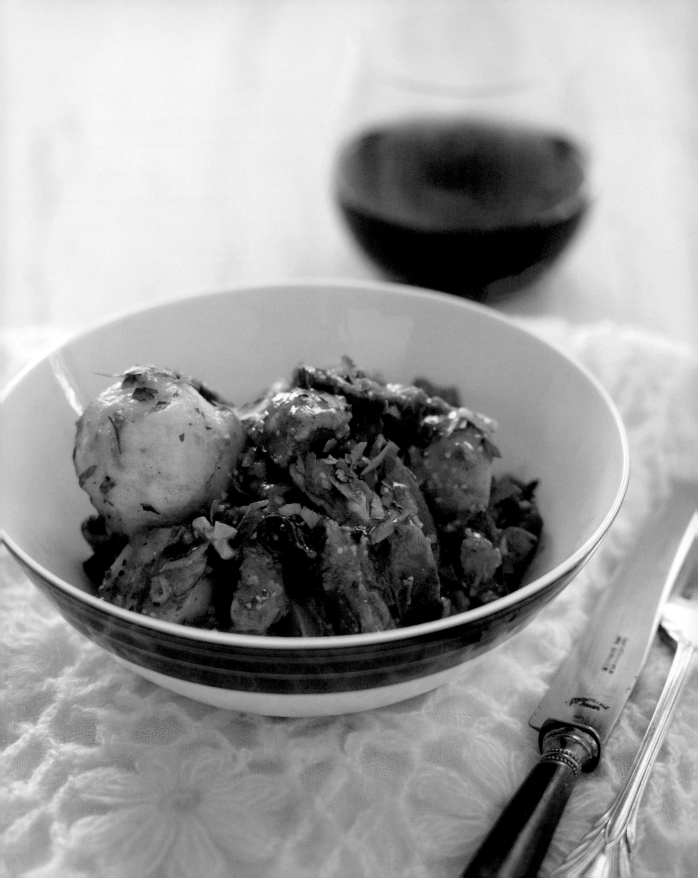

Beef and Bacon Casserole with Dumplings

SERVES 10

Dumplings are an old-fashioned favorite, but because they are normally wheat-based, they're off the menu for many people. Not anymore. Now you can enjoy a comforting casserole with lots of gravy, topped with plump wheat-free potato dumplings.

1. Preheat the oven to 280°F (140°C).

2. Place the cornstarch in a large bowl and season with salt and pepper. Add the beef, toss, and shake off any excess.

3. Heat 2 teaspoons of the oil in a Dutch oven over medium heat. Add the bacon and potatoes, and cook for 6 to 8 minutes, until the potatoes are golden and tender. Transfer to a bowl.

4. Heat 2 teaspoons of the oil in the Dutch oven. Add half of the beef and cook, stirring occasionally, for 2 minutes, or until browned all over. Transfer to a bowl. Repeat with the remaining oil and beef. Return the beef and the potato mixture to the pot.

5. Combine the brandy, mustard, cream, and stock, and pour into the pot. Bring to a boil over medium heat. Remove from the heat and season with salt and pepper. Cover and bake for 2 hours.

6. Meanwhile, place the potatoes in a large saucepan and cover with cold water. Bring to a boil and cook for 15 minutes, or until tender. Drain and set aside for 5 minutes. Return to the pan. Add the milk and butter, and mash until smooth. Sift the rice flour, cornstarch, and tapioca flour three times into a medium bowl (or mix with a whisk so they are well combined). Stir the flour mixture, cheese, and parsley into the potatoes and season to taste with additional salt and pepper. Shape into 12 dumplings.

7. Remove the Dutch oven from the oven, stir in the spinach, and top with the dumplings. Cover and bake for 20 minutes. Remove the lid and bake for 15 to 20 minutes, until the dumplings are golden and the beef is tender. Garnish with parsley and serve.

PER SERVING: 609 calories; 55 g protein; 23 g total fat; 9.7 g saturated fat; 36.9 g carbohydrates; 2.2 g fiber; 860 mg sodium

2 tablespoons cornstarch

Salt and freshly ground black pepper

2½ pounds (1.2 kg) boneless beef blade steak, cut into 1-inch (3 cm) cubes

6 teaspoons (30 ml) garlic-infused canola oil

½ pound (250 g) lean bacon slices, cut into thin strips

1½ pounds (700 g) new potatoes, cut in half

½ cup (125 ml) brandy

2 tablespoons whole grain mustard

½ cup (125 ml) light cream

1 cup (250 ml) onion-free beef stock (gluten-free if following a gluten-free diet), or to taste

4 cups (80 g) baby spinach leaves

DUMPLINGS

2 large red-skin potatoes, peeled

¾ cup (185 ml) low-fat milk, lactose-free milk, or suitable plant-based milk

3 tablespoons (40 g) butter

¾ cup (100 g) fine rice flour

½ cup (75 g) cornstarch

3 tablespoons tapioca flour

½ cup (40 g) grated Parmesan

2 tablespoons chopped flat-leaf parsley, plus additional for garnish

Salt and black pepper

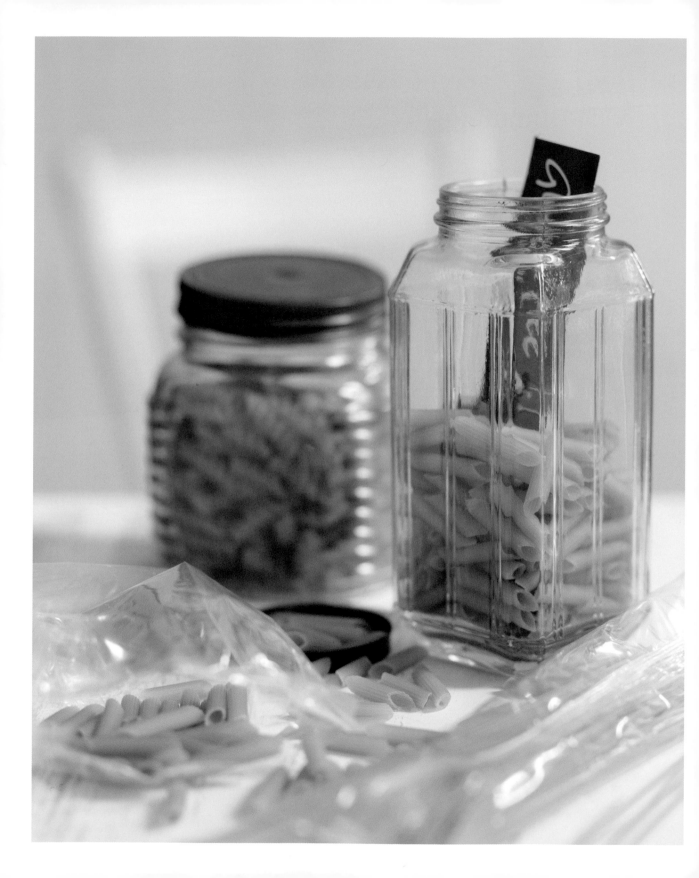

Pasta, Noodles, and Rice

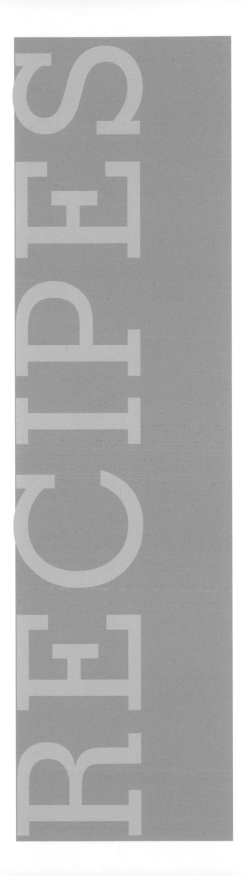

Pasta with Ricotta and Lemon

SERVES 6

People with lactose intolerance can still enjoy this delicious pasta dish—simply replace the ricotta with shredded buffalo mozzarella or *bocconcini*. The cheese won't melt in quite the same way as ricotta, but it will still result in a most enjoyable meal.

1. Cook the pasta in a large pot of boiling water until just tender, following the package instructions. Drain and return to the pot.

2. Combine the ricotta, spinach, parsley, grated lemon zest, and lemon juice in a bowl. Mix in the hot pasta. Season to taste with salt and pepper. Garnish with the additional lemon zest, if desired, and serve immediately.

PER SERVING: 335 calories; 7.9 g protein; 3.4 g total fat; 1.7 g saturated fat; 68.0 g carbohydrates; 0.3 g fiber; 53 mg sodium

1 pound (500 g) gluten-free pasta

1 cup (200 g) ricotta

3 cups (60 g) baby spinach leaves

¼ cup (15 g) chopped flat-leaf parsley

Grated zest of 1 lemon, plus additional thin strips of lemon zest for garnish, optional

3 tablespoons lemon juice

Salt and freshly ground black pepper

Tuscan Tuna Pasta

These days, there are so many varieties of gluten-free pasta available that you can enjoy this simple dish with any shape of pasta you like. For this recipe, look for sun-dried tomatoes packed in oil. If you must use the dry-packed variety, soak the tomatoes in warm water for 30 minutes before making the dressing; otherwise, they will be too tough.

1. Place the oil, crushed red pepper, and tomatoes in a jar and shake well to combine. Set aside for 1 hour.

2. Cook the pasta in a large pot of boiling water until just tender, following the package instructions. Drain and return to the pot. Stir in the oil mixture, tuna, olives, and half of the basil.

3. Divide the pasta among six bowls and top with the Parmesan and remaining basil.

PER SERVING: 469 calories; 18.5 g protein; 15.5 g total fat; 3.4 g saturated fat; 56.5 g carbohydrates; 13.1 g fiber; 337 mg sodium

2 tablespoons garlic-infused olive oil

1 teaspoon crushed red pepper

⅓ cup (100 g) sun-dried tomatoes packed in oil, drained and chopped

1 pound (500 g) gluten-free pasta

7 ounces (200 g) canned tuna in oil, drained and flaked

½ cup plus 2 tablespoons (100 g) chopped kalamata olives

½ cup (30 g) shredded basil

½ cup (40 g) grated Parmesan

Spinach and Pancetta Pasta

SERVES 6

Pancetta is unsmoked dried pork belly that has been salt-cured and spiced. It may be eaten raw but is often lightly panfried to enhance its depth of flavor. I find this makes a big difference, especially in simple dishes like this one.

1. Cook the pasta in a large pot of boiling water until just tender, following the package instructions. Drain and return to the pot. Stir in 1 tablespoon of the oil. Cover to keep warm.

2. Heat the remaining 1 tablespoon of oil in a large skillet. Add the pancetta, spinach, and pine nuts, and cook until the pine nuts are golden and the spinach has wilted. Add the pasta and Parmesan, and toss over medium heat until the cheese has melted. Season to taste with salt and pepper, and serve with an extra splash of the oil, if desired.

PER SERVING: 492 calories; 18.7 g protein; 16.7 g total fat; 5 g saturated fat; 66.9 g carbohydrates; 0.3 g fiber; 1,087 mg sodium

1 pound (500 g) gluten-free pasta

2 tablespoons garlic-infused olive oil, plus additional for serving, optional

8 ounces (225 g) thinly sliced lean pancetta

5 cups (100 g) baby spinach leaves

¼ cup (30 g) pine nuts

½ cup (40 g) grated Parmesan

Salt and freshly ground black pepper

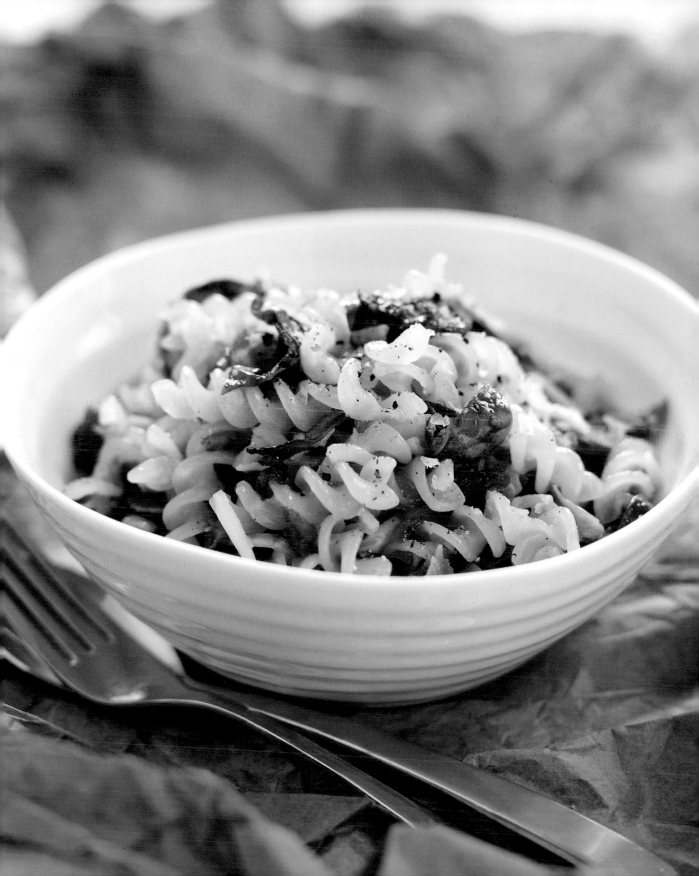

Chicken and Pepper Pilaf

SERVES 6 TO 8

I love the versatility of rice—it fits right in with so many different styles of cooking. Making a pilaf (also called *pilau*) involves heating rice in oil and then cooking it gently in stock or broth. Although the mix of whole spices gives this pilaf a wonderful depth of flavor, you can substitute 2 teaspoons of Chinese five-spice powder and 2 to 3 teaspoons of curry powder (gluten-free if necessary), though this will change the taste of the dish.

1. Rinse the rice under cold water until the water runs clear. Place the rice in a bowl, cover with cold water, and let soak for 20 minutes.

2. Combine the saffron and 1 tablespoon of hot water in a cup, then set aside to infuse.

3. Heat 2 tablespoons of the oil in a large skillet over medium-high heat. Add the chicken and celery, and cook, stirring regularly, for 5 to 6 minutes, until the chicken is golden brown and the celery has softened. Transfer to a plate.

4. Reduce the heat to medium-low. Add the remaining 1 tablespoon of oil, cinnamon, cardamom, cloves, star anise, curry leaves, ginger, and chile, and cook, stirring, for 1 minute, or until fragrant. Drain the rice and add to the pan, stirring to coat well in the spice mixture.

5. Increase the heat to high and add the saffron mixture, stock, and chicken. Bring to a boil, then reduce the heat to low and cook, covered, for 20 minutes, or until the rice is tender and the liquid has been absorbed. Remove the pan from the heat and stir in the bell peppers. Cover and set aside for about 10 minutes before serving. If possible, remove the whole spices before serving; otherwise, warn those eating the pilaf to avoid them.

PER SERVING (one eighth of recipe): 388 calories; 29.4 g protein; 10.9 g total fat; 2.4 g saturated fat; 42.1 g carbohydrates; 1.4 g fiber; 436 mg sodium

2 cups (400 g) basmati rice

Small pinch of saffron threads

3 tablespoons garlic-infused canola oil

1½ pounds (750 g) boneless skinless chicken breasts, sliced

2 stalks celery, cut into thin slices

1-inch (3 cm) piece cinnamon stick

2 green cardamom pods

2 cloves

1 star anise

20 fresh curry leaves

1 tablespoon chopped ginger

2 small red chile peppers, finely chopped

3 cups (750 ml) onion-free chicken stock (gluten-free if following a gluten-free diet)

½ red bell pepper, sliced

½ green bell pepper, sliced

½ yellow bell pepper, sliced

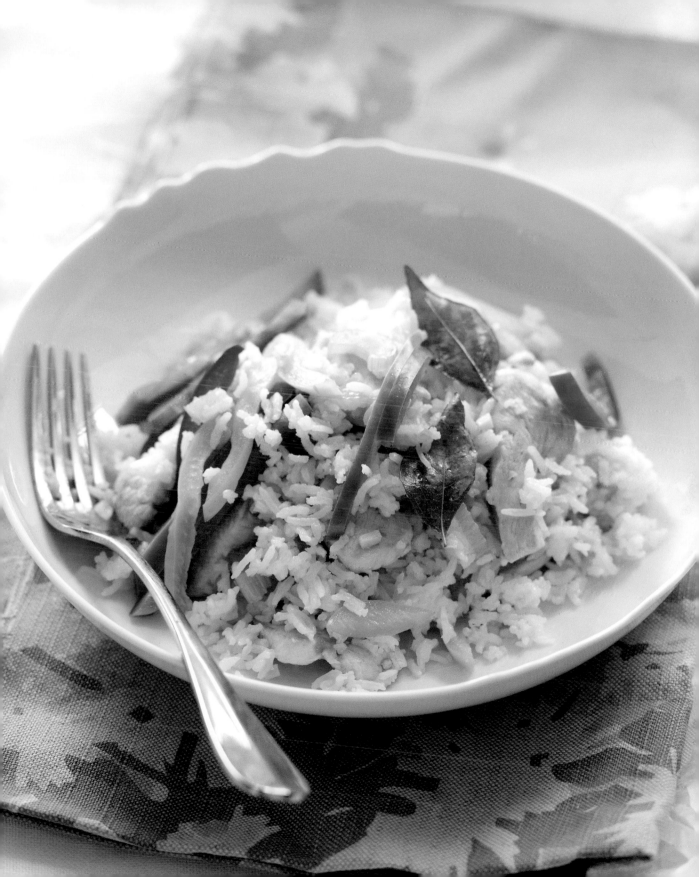

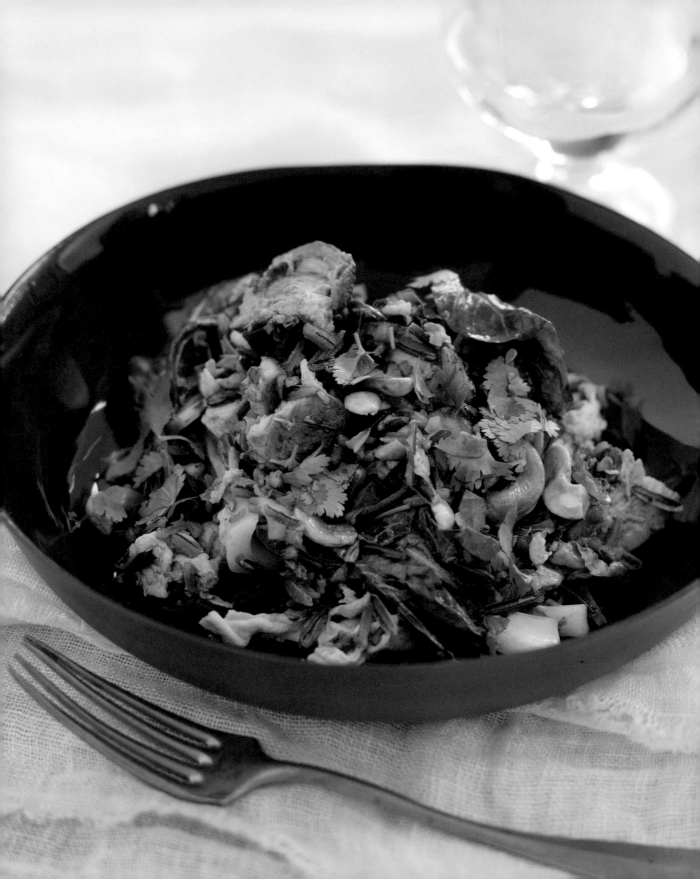

Chinese Chicken on Fried Wild Rice

SERVES 6

Wild rice looks and tastes sensational, and it makes a nice change from white rice. Here, its distinctive nutty flavor is enhanced by a handful of roasted peanuts.

1. Combine the soy sauce, ginger, garlic-infused oil, and five-spice powder in a small bowl. Place the chicken in a nonmetallic dish, pour in the marinade, and toss to coat. Cover and marinate in the fridge for 2 to 3 hours.

2. To start preparing the fried rice, place the rice in a medium saucepan and cover with 3¾ cups (900 ml) cold water. Bring to a boil and cook, covered, over medium heat for 45 minutes, or until tender and beginning to curl. Drain and set aside for 20 minutes to cool completely.

3. Preheat the oven to 350°F (180°C).

4. Spray a large nonstick skillet with cooking spray, add the chicken, and cook over medium-high heat for 2 minutes on each side. Transfer to a roasting pan and bake for 20 to 25 minutes, until cooked through, turning once. Remove from the oven and keep warm.

5. Meanwhile, heat 1 teaspoon of the peanut oil in a wok or large skillet. Add the peanuts, and cook, stirring frequently, until lightly toasted. Transfer to a plate. Heat the remaining oil in the pan. Add the eggs, and cook, stirring and breaking it up into pieces. Add the cooked wild rice, peanuts, and soy sauce, and cook, stirring regularly, for 2 to 3 minutes, until heated through. Remove from the heat. Stir in the cilantro and season to taste with salt and pepper.

6. Cut the chicken into ½-inch (1 cm) slices and toss with the fried rice. Divide among six plates, garnish with the additional cilantro, and serve immediately with the steamed Asian greens.

PER SERVING (including ½ cup steamed Asian greens): 522 calories; 57.4 g protein; 18.7 g total fat; 4.2 g saturated fat; 28.2 g carbohydrates; 6.0 g fiber; 856 mg sodium

3 tablespoons soy sauce (gluten-free if following a gluten-free diet)

2 teaspoons grated ginger

1 tablespoon garlic-infused canola oil

1 teaspoon Chinese five-spice powder

Four 6-ounce (170 g) boneless skinless chicken breasts

FRIED WILD RICE

1¼ cups (200 g) wild rice

2 teaspoons peanut oil

½ cup (75 g) roasted peanuts, roughly chopped

2 eggs, lightly beaten

1 tablespoon soy sauce (gluten-free if following a gluten-free diet)

2 tablespoons coarsely chopped cilantro, plus additional for garnish

Salt and freshly ground black pepper

Steamed Asian greens

Singapore Noodles

SERVES 4

If you have celiac disease, use gluten-free curry powder, soy sauce, and stock for this recipe. Those following the low-FODMAP diet who do not have celiac disease don't have to take this precaution as the amount of wheat present should not cause any problems.

1. Cover the vermicelli noodles with boiling water and let soak until soft. Rinse with cold water, drain, and set aside.

2. Heat both oils in a wok or skillet over high heat until very hot but not smoking. Add the ginger and chile, and stir-fry for 30 seconds. Reduce the heat to medium-high. Add the shrimp and squid, and stir-fry for 1 minute. Add the bean sprouts and pork, and stir-fry for an additional 2 minutes.

3. Make a well in the center of the mixture. Pour in the beaten eggs, and cook, stirring enough to lightly scramble.

4. Add the curry powder, soy sauce, brown sugar, chicken stock, and cooked noodles, and stir until all the liquid has been absorbed. Season to taste with salt and pepper. Divide among four bowls, sprinkle with chives, and serve.

PER SERVING: 443 calories; 55.3 g protein; 18.8 g total fat; 3.3 g saturated fat; 12.2 g carbohydrates; 0.8 g fiber; 976 mg sodium

1 cup (50 g) rice vermicelli

2 tablespoons garlic-infused canola oil

2 tablespoons sesame oil

1 teaspoon grated ginger

1 small red chile, finely chopped

4 ounces (125 g) peeled raw shrimp, deveined

5 small squid hoods, cleaned and thinly sliced

1 cup (80 g) bean sprouts

8 ounces (225 g) pork loin chops, thinly sliced

2 eggs, beaten

3 to 4 teaspoons curry powder (gluten-free if following a gluten-free diet)

1 tablespoon soy sauce (gluten-free if following a gluten-free diet)

2 teaspoons brown sugar

3 tablespoons onion-free chicken stock (gluten-free if following a gluten-free diet)

Salt and freshly ground black pepper

Chopped chives

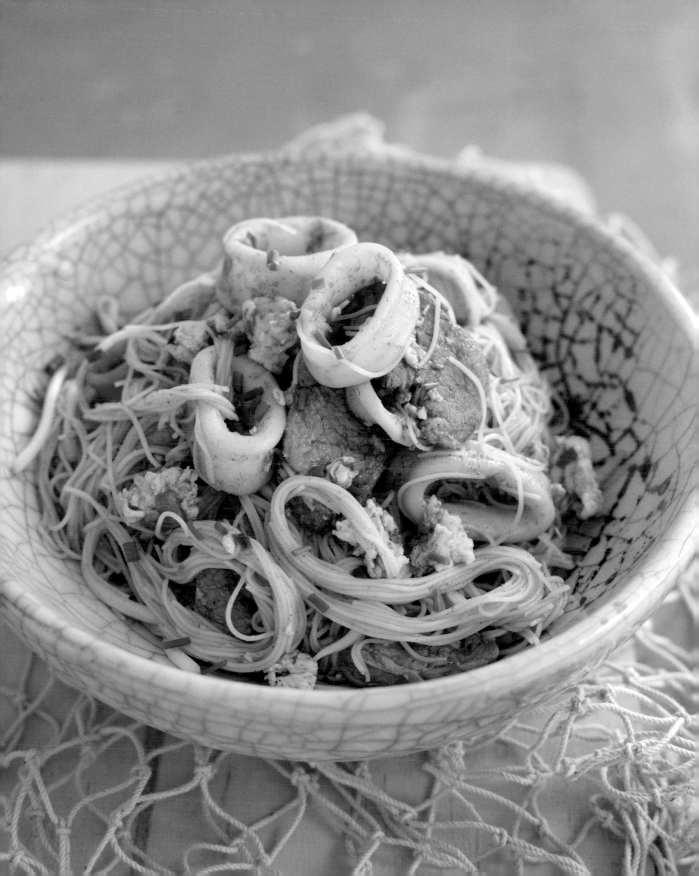

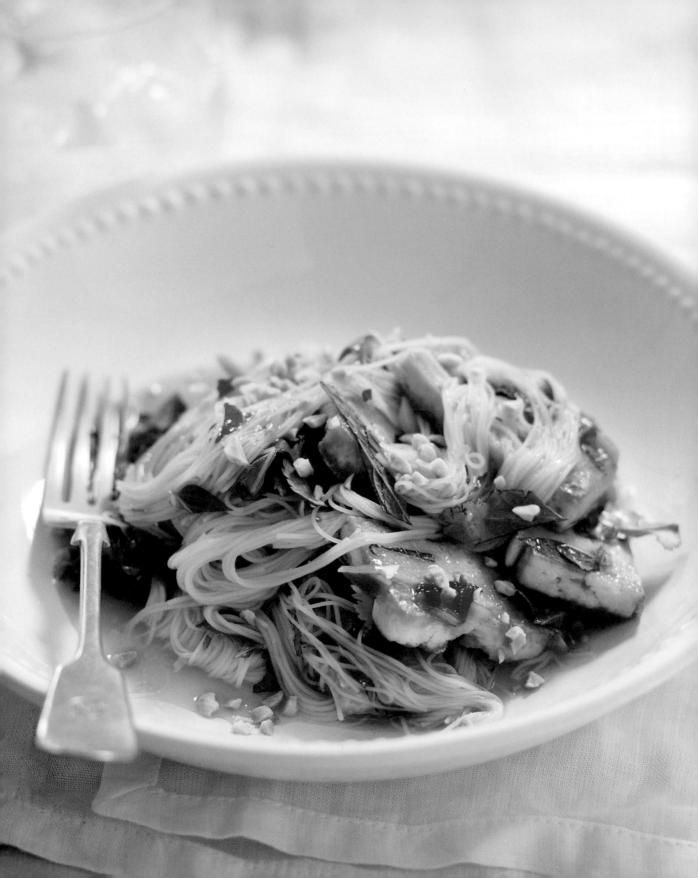

Thai-Inspired Stir-Fry with Tofu and Vermicelli

SERVES 4

Many noodles, such as hokkien, udon, and egg noodles, are made from wheat and are, therefore, not suitable for people on the low-FODMAP diet. However, all is not lost: Rice vermicelli is available in a range of thicknesses, and glass noodles (made from mungbeans) and 100% buckwheat soba noodles can also be found in grocery stores and Asian markets. Tofu is a great vegetarian protein source that is tolerated by many on the low-FODMAP diet. Assess your individual tolerance.

1. Cover the vermicelli noodles with boiling water to soak until soft. Rinse with cool water and drain. Set aside. Combine the sweet chili sauce, fish sauce, and ginger in a small bowl.

2. To make the sauce, mix the cornstarch and about 2 tablespoons of the warm water in a cup to form a paste. Add the remaining water and mix well. Pour into the sweet chili sauce mixture and stir until well combined.

3. Heat the oil in a medium skillet over medium-high heat. Add the tofu and cook, turning once, for 3 minutes, or until golden brown. Add the sauce and stir gently until the sauce thickens. Stir in the noodles, cilantro, and mint. Garnish with the crushed peanuts and serve immediately.

PER SERVING: 544 calories; 19.8 g protein; 15.2 g total fat; 2.3 g saturated fat; 73.3 g carbohydrates; 11 g fiber; 1,058 mg sodium

8 ounces (250 g) rice vermicelli

⅔ cup (160 ml) garlic-free sweet chili sauce

2 tablespoons fish sauce, or 1 teaspoon soy sauce (gluten-free if following a gluten-free diet)

2 teaspoons grated ginger

1 tablespoon cornstarch

1 cup (250 ml) warm water

1 teaspoon garlic-infused oil

1 teaspoon peanut oil

One 14-ounce (400 g) package firm tofu, pressed if desired, cut into thick slices

¼ cup chopped cilantro, packed

1 cup (50 g) chopped mint

2 tablespoons crushed peanuts

Stir-Fried Pork with Chile and Cilantro

SERVES 4

This simple stir-fry recipe also works well with other proteins substituted for the pork: beef, chicken, shrimp, tofu, or tempeh would all be fine.

1. Place the chile, sherry, cornstarch, and brown sugar in a small jar and shake to combine well.

2. Heat 1 teaspoon of the oil in a large wok or skillet over high heat. Add half of the pork strips and toss just until no longer pink. Transfer the pork to a plate. Repeat with the remaining pork strips.

3. Heat the remaining 1 teaspoon of oil in the wok or pan. Add the carrot and celery, and stir-fry for 3 minutes, or until tender but starting to crisp around the edges. Add the chile mixture and pork strips, and stir-fry for another 2 minutes. Remove from the heat, stir in the cilantro, and serve immediately with the rice.

PER SERVING (including ½ cup cooked rice): 374 calories; 46.4 g protein; 5.9 g total fat; 1.5 g saturated fat; 30.7 g carbohydrates; 1.4 g fiber; 138 mg sodium

1 small red chile, thinly sliced

2 tablespoons dry sherry, or an additional 1 tablespoon brown sugar

2 teaspoons cornstarch

2 teaspoons brown sugar

2 teaspoons sesame oil

1 pound (500 g) boneless pork chops, cut into thin strips

2 carrots, peeled and finely sliced on the diagonal

2 stalks celery, finely sliced on the diagonal

⅓ cup (20 g) cilantro leaves

Cooked white rice

Risotto Milanese

SERVES 6

This simple, traditionally flavored risotto may be enjoyed as a main course, but its mild flavor also makes it a perfect accompaniment to meat and poultry dishes. I particularly like it with slow-cooked meat, so tender it's falling off the bone.

1. Heat the oil in a large saucepan. Add the saffron and stir over medium heat for 2 minutes. Add the rice and stir for 1 to 2 minutes, until the rice is well coated in the saffron mixture.

2. Pour the stock into a medium saucepan over low heat and keep at a low simmer. Add the wine to the rice and cook until absorbed. Pour in 1 cup (250 ml) of the heated stock and cook, stirring, until absorbed. Add the remaining stock ½ cup (125 ml) at a time, reserving the last ½ cup (125 ml) of stock for later. Stir in the Parmesan and parsley. Pour in the reserved stock, stirring until completely absorbed. Taste, season with salt and pepper, and serve.

PER SERVING: 384 calories; 10.5 g protein; 6.3 g total fat; 2.2 g saturated fat; 68.9 g carbohydrates; 0.8 g fiber; 1,386 mg sodium

1 tablespoon garlic-infused olive oil

1 teaspoon saffron threads

2½ cups (500 g) arborio rice

8 cups (2 liters) onion-free vegetable stock (gluten-free if following a gluten-free diet)

½ cup (125 ml) dry white wine, or additional vegetable stock

½ cup (40 g) grated Parmesan

¼ cup (15 g) chopped flat-leaf parsley

Salt and freshly ground black pepper

Tomato Chicken Risotto

SERVES 6

There's something very comforting about a bowl of creamy risotto, especially when it's homemade. This version is free of onions and garlic, so it is suitable for people following the low-FODMAP diet.

1. Heat 1 tablespoon of the oil in a small skillet over medium-high heat. Add the chicken and cook, tossing regularly, until lightly golden. Remove from the heat and set aside.

2. Pour the stock into a saucepan over low heat and keep at a low simmer.

3. Heat the remaining 1 tablespoon of oil in a large heavy-bottomed saucepan. Add the rice and stir for 1 to 2 minutes until the rice is well coated with oil. Pour in the wine and cook until absorbed. Add 1 cup (250 ml) of the heated stock and cook, stirring, until absorbed. Add all but ½ cup (125 ml) of the remaining stock, ½ cup (125 ml) at a time, cooking and stirring between each addition until the stock is absorbed.

4. Add the chicken, spinach, tomatoes, Parmesan, and parsley, and stir until well combined. Pour in the reserved stock, stirring until completely absorbed. Season with salt and pepper, and serve garnished with extra parsley.

PER SERVING: 508 calories; 25.2 g protein; 13.1 g total fat; 3.5 g saturated fat; 69.3 g carbohydrates; 1.3 g fiber; 1,527 mg sodium

2 tablespoons garlic-infused olive oil

Two 6-ounce (170 g) boneless skinless chicken breasts, sliced

8 cups (2 liters) onion-free chicken stock (gluten-free if following a gluten-free diet)

2½ cups (500 g) arborio rice

½ cup (125 ml) dry white wine, optional

2 cups (40 g) baby spinach leaves

1 cup (220 g) canned chopped tomatoes

½ cup (40 g) grated Parmesan

¼ cup (15 g) chopped flat-leaf parsley, plus additional leaves for garnish

Salt and freshly ground black pepper

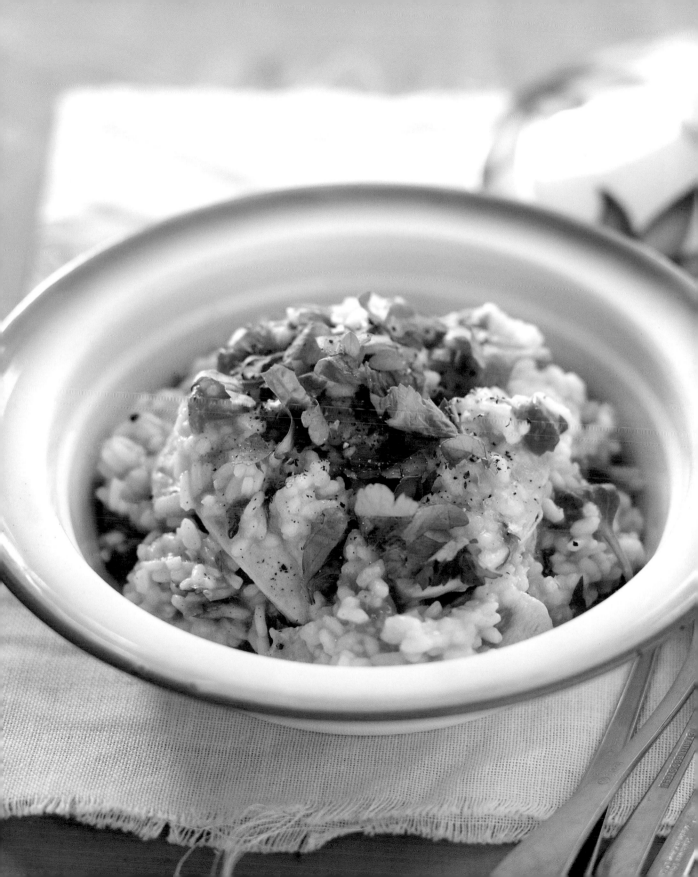

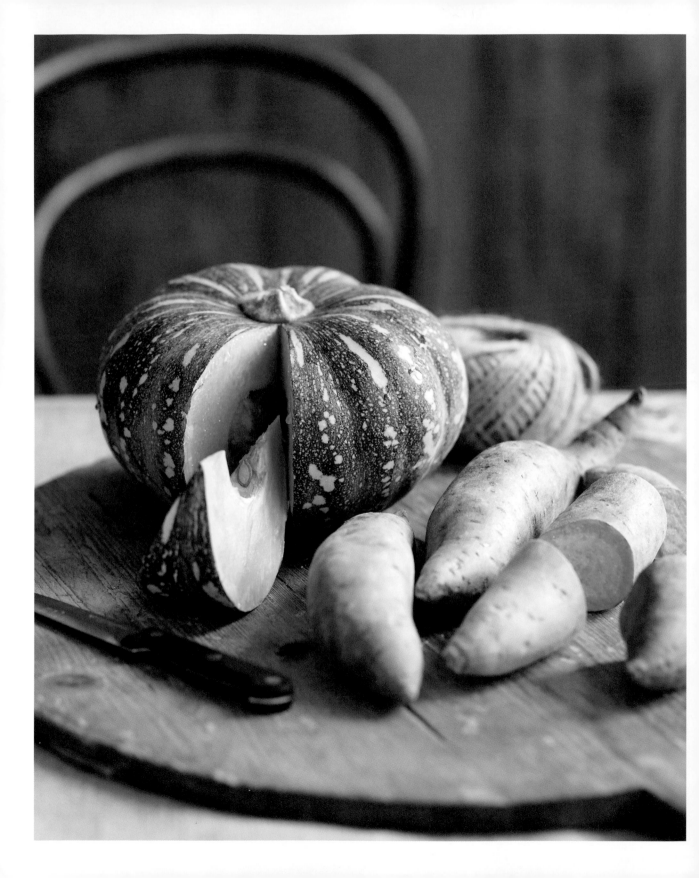

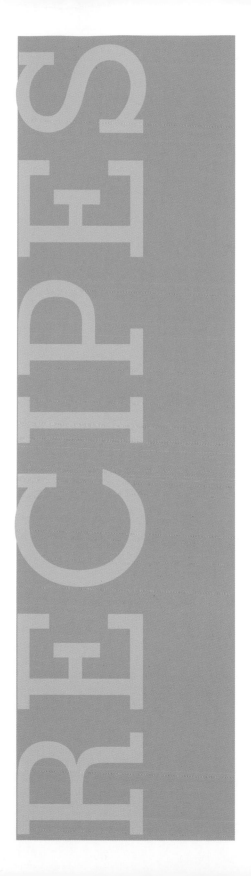

Entrées

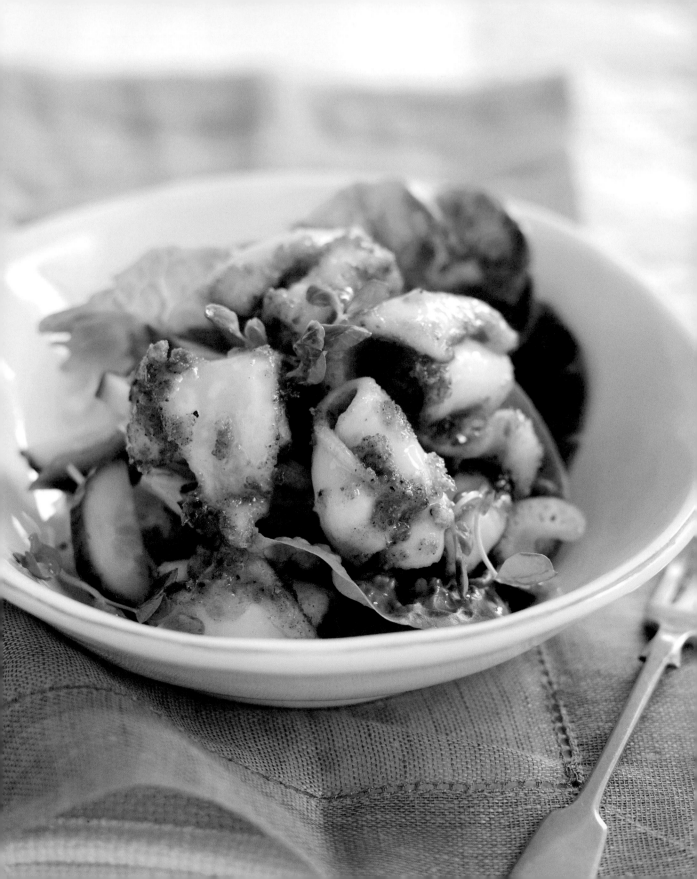

Paprika Calamari with Garden Salad

SERVES 4

Calamari looks so inviting to eat when it is curled up, as it is in this recipe. The trick is to use thick pieces of squid. Cut them open, then with the inside of the squid facing up, cut in a criss-cross pattern. This will ensure the calamari curls beautifully during cooking.

1. Cut the squid bodies down the long sides to make two large pieces (if using large squid, cut them into quarters). With a sharp knife, cut the squid pieces in a ½-inch (1 cm) crisscross pattern, taking care not to cut all the way through. Pat dry with paper towels.

2. Combine the salt, pepper, paprika, and cornstarch in a large bowl, add the squid pieces, and toss to coat. Cover and refrigerate for 3 to 4 hours.

3. To prepare the salad, combine the lettuce, cucumber, celery, bell pepper, and snow pea shoots in a large salad bowl.

4. To make the dressing, place the oil, lemon juice, and brown sugar in a small screw-top jar and shake well to combine. Season to taste with salt.

5. Preheat the grill to hot, or heat a skillet or ridged grill pan over high heat. Brush the grill or pan with oil. Add the squid, scored-side down, and cook for 2 to 3 minutes. Turn and cook for another 1 to 2 minutes, until the squid has become an opaque white color throughout.

6. Divide the salad among four bowls or plates, and drizzle with the dressing. Arrange the calamari on top and serve warm.

PER SERVING: 223 calories; 22.3 g protein; 8.6 g total fat; 1.6 g saturated fat; 13.5 g carbohydrates; 1.6 g fiber; 405 mg sodium

4 large or 8 regular squid bodies, cleaned

½ teaspoon salt

½ teaspoon finely ground black pepper

1 teaspoon paprika

⅓ cup (50 g) cornstarch

Olive oil

GARDEN SALAD

1 small head romaine lettuce, roughly chopped

½ large cucumber, halved lengthwise and sliced

2 stalks celery, thinly sliced

½ green bell pepper, seeded and sliced

1 cup (50 g) snow pea shoots

DRESSING

2 tablespoons garlic-infused olive oil

1½ tablespoons lemon juice

½ teaspoon brown sugar

Salt

Chili Salmon with Cilantro Salad

SERVES 4

Salmon is one of the richest sources of omega-3 fats, which are important for the prevention of heart disease. In particular, salmon contains a type of fat called DHA, which is important for brain development. The sweet chili sauce is a simple, flavorful addition to this delicious and nutritious food from the sea.

1. Line a broiler pan with foil and set an oven rack 5 inches from the broiler element. Place the salmon fillets on the pan, skin-side up, and broil for 1 to 2 minutes, until the skin becomes crispy. Turn the fillets over and brush ¾ teaspoon of the sweet chili sauce over each. Season with salt and pepper. Broil for an additional 3 to 4 minutes, or until cooked to your liking.

2. Meanwhile, to make the salad, mix together the lettuce, cucumber, celery, bell pepper, and cilantro in a large bowl. Combine the chile, lime juice, rice vinegar, fish sauce, and brown sugar in a small bowl and pour over the salad. Serve with the salmon.

PER SERVING: 353 calories; 40.3 g protein; 17.3 g total fat; 4.4 g saturated fat; 8.7 g carbohydrates; 2.0 g fiber; 852 mg sodium

Four 5½-ounce (160 g) salmon fillets, skin on, pin bones removed

1 tablespoon garlic-free sweet chili sauce

Salt and freshly ground black pepper

CILANTRO SALAD

5 cups (150 g) roughly chopped lettuce leaves

½ large cucumber, halved lengthwise and sliced

2 stalks celery, thinly sliced on the diagonal

½ green bell pepper, thinly sliced

½ cup (25 g) firmly packed chopped cilantro

½ small red chile, finely chopped

2 tablespoons lime juice

1 tablespoon rice vinegar

2 tablespoons fish sauce

2 tablespoons brown sugar

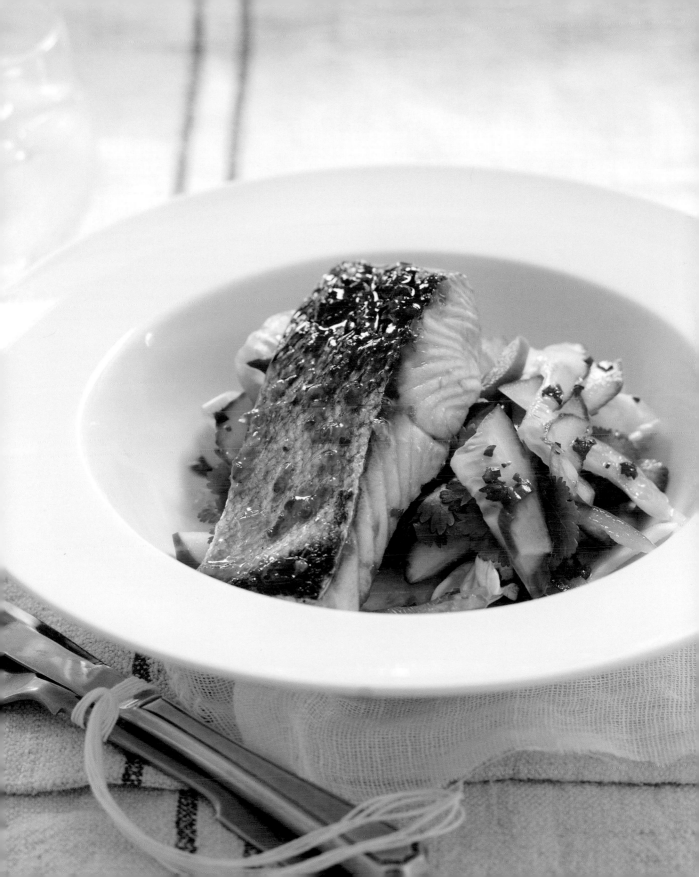

Dukkah-Crusted Snapper

SERVES 4

Dukkah is an Egyptian spice blend typically made with sesame seeds, nuts, ground coriander, and cumin. I like to serve these fillets with gently spiced rice, made by stirring a little butter, ½ teaspoon ground cumin, and 1 tablespoon finely chopped cilantro into cooked basmati rice, but plain rice is also delicious.

1. To make the dukkah, preheat the oven to 350°F (180°C) and line a baking sheet with parchment paper. Spread out the almonds and pine nuts on the baking sheet and bake for 5 minutes, or until golden. Cool to room temperature. Place all the nuts and spices in a food processor and pulse until fine crumbs are formed. Reserve 4 tablespoons to serve, and transfer the rest to a plate.

2. Brush the fish fillets all over with the oil, then press into the dukkah to coat both sides. Heat a ridged grill pan or a cast-iron skillet over medium-high heat. Add the fish and cook for 3 to 4 minutes on each side, until just cooked. Sprinkle with the cilantro and the reserved dukkah. Serve with the basmati rice and lemon wedges.

PER SERVING (including ½ cup cooked white rice): 536 calories; 48.4 g protein; 26.2 g total fat; 2.6 g saturated fat; 26.4 g carbohydrates; 0.8 g fiber; 174 mg sodium

DUKKAH

½ cup (75 g) blanched almonds

¼ cup (30 g) pine nuts

1 teaspoon ground coriander

1 teaspoon cumin seeds

1 teaspoon sesame seeds

½ teaspoon chili powder

Four 7-ounce (200 g) snapper fillets (ideally about 1-inch/ 3 cm thick), or other lean fish

2 tablespoons canola oil

Cilantro leaves

Cooked basmati rice

Lemon wedges

Balsamic Sesame Swordfish

Swordfish is a meaty fish, purchased as steaks, so there is no wastage. This recipe also works very well with tuna steaks, tempeh, or well-pressed tofu.

1. Combine the balsamic vinegar, soy sauce, and brown sugar in a nonmetallic bowl. Add the swordfish steaks and turn to coat in the marinade. Cover and refrigerate for 3 to 4 hours, turning regularly.

2. Preheat the oven to 450°F (230°C). Line a large baking sheet with parchment paper.

3. Place the swordfish steaks on the baking sheet, reserving the marinade, and bake for 10 minutes. Turn the steaks over and baste with the marinade. Sprinkle with sesame seeds and bake for an additional 5 to 10 minutes, until cooked through. Serve with the steamed Asian greens.

PER SERVING (including ½ cup steamed Asian greens): 480 calories; 56.3 g protein; 25 g total fat; 6.1 g saturated fat; 9.6 g carbohydrates; 4.3 g fiber; 699 mg sodium

3 tablespoons balsamic vinegar

2 tablespoons soy sauce (gluten-free if following a gluten-free diet)

2 tablespoons brown sugar

4 large swordfish steaks

1½ tablespoons sesame seeds

Steamed Asian greens

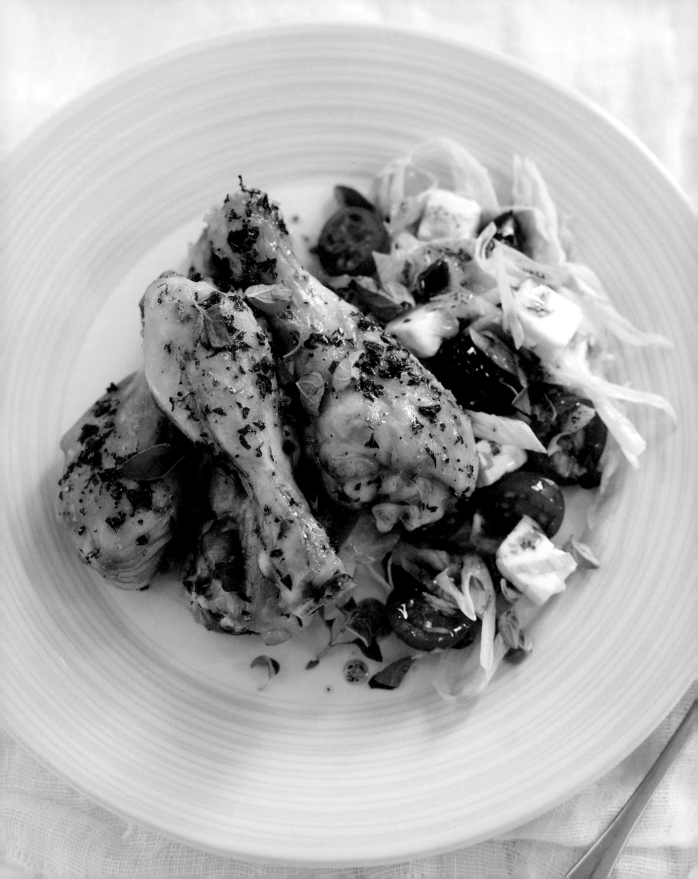

Lemon-Oregano Chicken Drumsticks

SERVES 6

These delicious drumsticks are so easy to prepare and wonderfully versatile—enjoy them as a main meal, as finger food at a party, or packed into a picnic hamper.

1. Use a small knife to pierce the chicken evenly all over.

2. Combine the oregano, lemon zest, and oil in a large bowl. Add the chicken, season with salt and pepper, and toss to coat. Cover and refrigerate for 3 to 4 hours, turning regularly.

3. Preheat the oven to 450°F (230°C). Line two baking sheets with parchment paper.

4. Place the drumsticks on the sheets and bake for 10 to 15 minutes, until golden brown and cooked through

5. Meanwhile, to make the salad, place the lettuce, tomatoes, olives, and feta in a large bowl and gently toss. Place the oil and vinegar in a small screw-top jar and shake well to combine. Pour over the salad and briefly toss. Serve with the chicken, garnished with the additional oregano.

PER SERVING: 498 calories; 53.6 g protein; 30.1 g total fat; 9.4 g saturated fat; 3.5 g carbohydrates; 0.5 g fiber; 560 mg sodium

18 skinless chicken drumsticks

¼ cup (15 g) finely chopped oregano, plus additional for garnish

1 tablespoon finely grated lemon zest

2 tablespoons extra virgin olive oil

Salt and freshly ground black pepper

GREEK SALAD

2 cups (120 g) shredded iceberg lettuce

12 cherry tomatoes, cut in half

½ cup (75 g) pitted kalamata olives

4 ounces (125 g) feta, cut into ½-inch (1 cm) cubes

2 tablespoons olive oil

2 teaspoons balsamic vinegar

Chicken with Maple-Mustard Sauce

SERVES 4

The unusual combination of maple syrup and mustard works brilliantly in this simple and delicious chicken dish.

1. Heat the oil in a large skillet over medium-low heat. Add the chicken and cook for 3 to 5 minutes on each side, until just cooked and golden brown. Remove from the pan. Cover and let rest while you make the sauce.

2. For the sauce, combine the cornstarch and a little of the chicken stock to form a paste. Gradually pour in the remaining stock, stirring well to ensure there are no lumps. Add the maple syrup, mustard, thyme, pepper, and cream.

3. Pour the sauce into the skillet and stir over medium-high heat for 3 to 5 minutes, until the sauce thickens. Return the chicken to the pan and toss in the sauce for 1 to 2 minutes, until heated through. Season to taste with salt, then serve immediately.

PER SERVING: 372 calories; 43.9 g protein; 15.9 g total fat; 4.7 g saturated fat; 13.7 g carbohydrates; 0.5 g fiber; 385 mg sodium

2 tablespoons garlic-infused canola oil

Four 6-ounce (170 g) boneless skinless chicken breasts

MAPLE-MUSTARD SAUCE

1 tablespoon cornstarch

1 cup (250 ml) onion-free chicken stock (gluten-free if following a gluten-free diet)

3 tablespoons pure maple syrup

1 tablespoon whole grain mustard

1 tablespoon chopped thyme

½ teaspoon freshly ground black pepper

2 tablespoons light whipping cream

Salt

Chicken with Herb Rösti

SERVES 6

Rösti are Swiss potato cakes with a crisp golden crust. They work best when the cooked potatoes are left to cool completely before being peeled and grated. This recipe makes four individual rösti; however, one large one can be made by cooking the mixture in a medium skillet. Rösti also make a great vegetarian meal, especially when topped with a poached egg and served with steamed vegetables.

1. Place the tarragon, olive oil, pepper, and cornstarch in a small screw-top jar and shake well to combine. Brush all over the chicken breasts. Cover and refrigerate for 1 to 2 hours.

2. To make the rösti, place the potatoes in a large saucepan, cover with cold water, and bring to a boil. Reduce the heat and simmer for 10 minutes. Drain. Let cool completely.

3. Peel the potatoes, then grate the flesh into a large bowl. Add the herbs and melted butter, and season to taste. Divide the mixture into six equal portions. Form each portion into a ball, then gently press flat with your hand to create a flat patty.

4. Heat the vegetable oil in a large nonstick skillet over medium heat. Add the rösti and cook for 10 to 15 minutes, until the bottom is crisp and golden. Flip with a spatula and cook for an additional 10 minutes, or until cooked through and golden brown.

5. Heat a large nonstick skillet sprayed with cooking spray over high heat and cook the chicken for 3 to 4 minutes on each side, until cooked through. Let the chicken rest for a few minutes.

6. Return the pan to medium-high heat. Add the stock and red wine, and bring to a simmer. Add the chicken and heat through for 2 minutes. Serve immediately with the herb rösti, steamed carrots, and a spoonful of mustard.

PER SERVING: 524 calories; 53.5 g protein; 26.2 g total fat; 12.2 g saturated fat; 16.4 g carbohydrates; 3.8 g fiber; 338 mg sodium

1 tablespoon finely chopped tarragon

1 tablespoon olive oil

2 tablespoons freshly ground black pepper

2 teaspoons cornstarch

Six 6-ounce (170 g) boneless skinless chicken breasts

HERB RÖSTI

4 large red-skin potatoes, such as Pontiac

2 tablespoons chopped flat-leaf parsley

6 sage leaves, chopped

8 tablespoons (115 g) butter, melted

Salt and freshly ground black pepper

2 tablespoons vegetable oil

½ cup (125 ml) onion-free beef stock (gluten-free if following a gluten-free diet)

⅓ cup (80 ml) red wine, or additional onion-free beef stock

Steamed baby carrots

Whole grain mustard

Prosciutto Chicken with Sage Polenta

SERVES 4

The creamy polenta is enhanced by the distinctive flavor of sage, providing a delicious base for the chicken. If you are unable to purchase prosciutto, bacon will work just as well.

1. Preheat the oven to 350°F (180°C) and line a baking sheet with parchment paper.

2. Wrap each chicken breast in a slice of prosciutto and secure with a toothpick. Place on the baking sheet and bake for 20 minutes, or until the chicken is cooked through and the prosciutto is crisp.

3. Meanwhile, to make the sage polenta, heat the milk and oil in a medium saucepan until almost boiling. Add the cornmeal and stir until the mixture boils. Reduce the heat to low and cook, stirring constantly, for an additional 3 to 5 minutes until the polenta is cooked (it should be the texture of smooth mashed potatoes). Stir in the sage and season with salt and pepper.

4. Spoon the polenta onto four warm plates and top with the prosciutto chicken. Sprinkle with additional sage leaves and serve.

PER SERVING: 505 calories; 66.8 g protein; 14.7 g total fat; 4.4 g saturated fat; 25.9 g carbohydrates; 0.6 g fiber; 374 mg sodium

Four 6-ounce (170 g) boneless skinless chicken breasts

4 slices prosciutto

SAGE POLENTA

3 cups (750 ml) low-fat milk, lactose-free milk, or suitable plant-based milk

2 tablespoons garlic-infused olive oil

²/₃ cup (85 g) cornmeal

2 tablespoons sage leaves, torn if large, plus additional for garnish

Salt and freshly ground black pepper

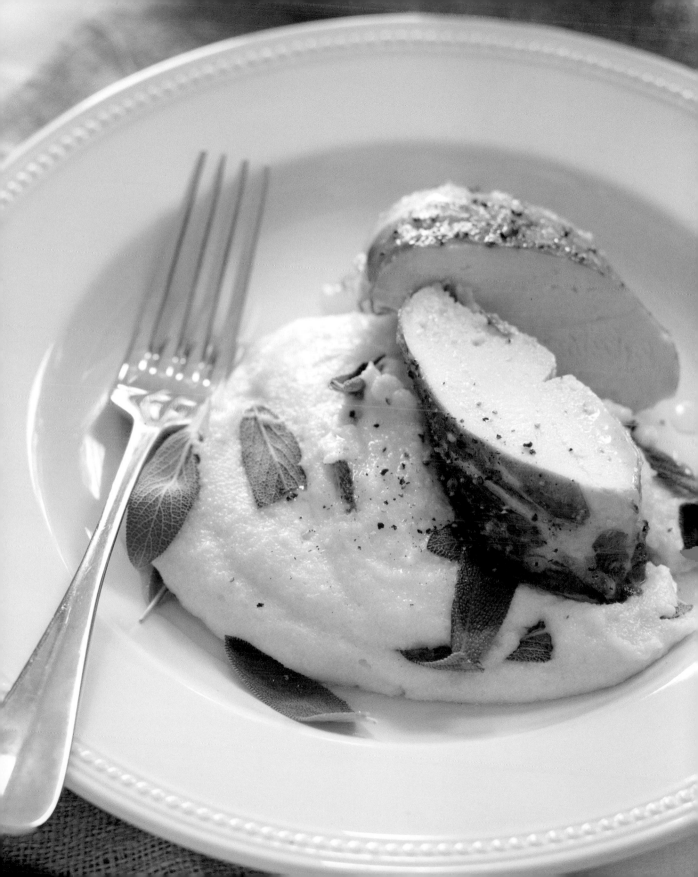

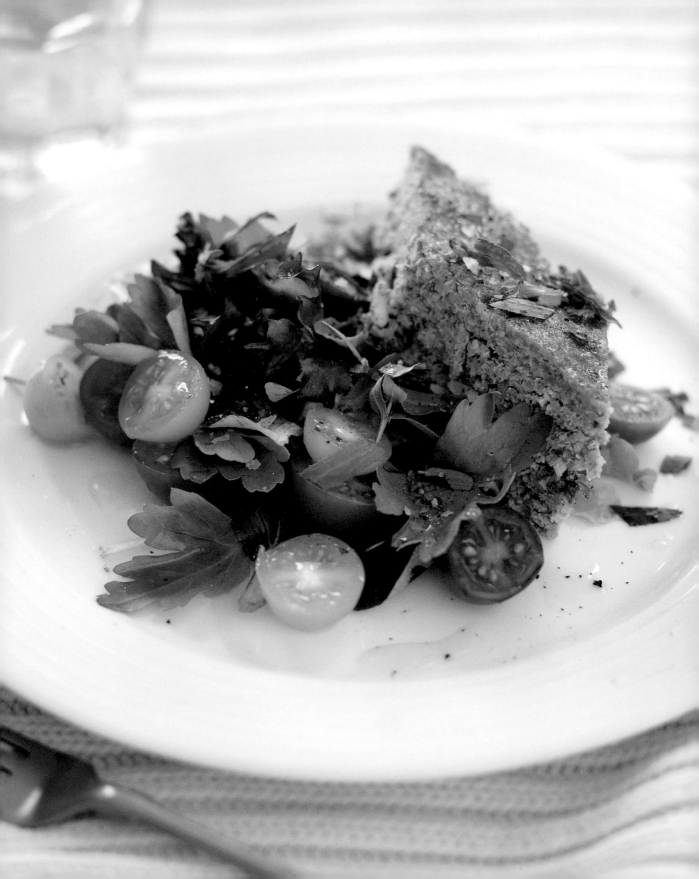

Chicken Kibbeh

SERVES 8 TO 10

Kibbeh is a Middle Eastern dish traditionally made with cracked wheat (bulgur) and pine nuts. This recipe uses quinoa, a wheat-free alternative to bulgur with a similar texture. Unless you are feeding a crowd you will have leftovers, but don't worry—it freezes well!

1. Preheat the oven to 350°F (180°C). Grease a 9 x 13-inch (25 x 30 cm) rimmed baking sheet and line with parchment paper.

2. Bring a medium saucepan of water to a boil and add the quinoa. Stir, then bring back to a boil. Cook for 10 to 12 minutes, until just tender. Drain and rinse under cold water, then drain again.

3. To make the filling, combine the pine nuts, tomatoes, cinnamon, parsley, and lemon zest in a small bowl.

4. Place the cooked quinoa, chicken, oil, tarragon, allspice, and tahini in a bowl and mix until well combined. Season to taste with salt and pepper. Divide into two portions. Press half of the mixture into the prepared baking sheet and cover evenly with the filling. Top with the remaining kibbeh mixture, spreading it evenly over the filling.

5. Bake for 50 to 60 minutes, until cooked through—a toothpick inserted into the center should come out clean. Remove and let rest for 5 to 10 minutes before cutting into squares. Garnish with the extra tarragon leaves and serve with the salad.

PER SERVING (one tenth of recipe, including 1 cup of salad):
298 calories; 23 g protein; 18.9 g total fat; 3.6 g saturated fat; 8.3 g carbohydrates; 2.6 g fiber; 94 mg sodium

1 cup (170 g) quinoa

FILLING

½ cup (80 g) pine nuts, toasted

3 small tomatoes, finely chopped

1 teaspoon ground cinnamon

1 cup (30 g) chopped flat-leaf parsley

1 teaspoon grated lemon zest

2 pounds (1 kg) ground chicken

2 tablespoons garlic-infused olive oil

3 tablespoons finely chopped tarragon, plus additional leaves for garnish

2 teaspoons ground allspice

2 tablespoons tahini

Salt and freshly ground black pepper

Garden Salad (page 163)

Roast Pork with Almond Stuffing

SERVES 8

Natural, or unblanched, almond flour has a great rustic texture, and it is a perfect flavor complement to the roast pork. If you can find it, you may substitute chestnut flour, which is made from coarsely ground chestnuts. It may be hard to find in supermarkets, so your best bet is to look for it in gourmet delis and Italian specialty stores.

1. Preheat the oven to 425°F (220°C).

2. Combine the almond flour, bread crumbs, herbs, and brown sugar in a bowl. Season with salt and pepper. Stir in the balsamic vinegar.

3. Open up the pork on a clean surface and spoon the stuffing along the center. Roll up the pork around the filling and tie it with kitchen string at 1-inch (2 cm) intervals.

4. Transfer the pork to a roasting pan and roast for 25 minutes. Reduce the temperature to 375°F (190°C) and roast for another hour. Transfer the pork to a plate and cover with foil. Let rest for 20 minutes. Remove the foil and cut the pork into slices. Garnish with the additional sage leaves and serve with the roasted vegetables and steamed zucchini flowers, if desired.

Scant ¾ cup (75 g) natural almond meal or chestnut flour

1½ cups (110 g) fresh gluten-free bread crumbs (made from day-old bread)

⅓ cup (10 g) chopped flat-leaf parsley

2 tablespoons chopped sage, plus additional leaves for garnish

3 tablespoons brown sugar

Salt and freshly ground black pepper

3 tablespoons balsamic vinegar

4-pound (1.8 kg) boneless center-cut pork loin, butterflied for stuffing

Roasted vegetables, such as potatoes, carrots, and parsnips

Steamed zucchini flowers, optional

PER SERVING (including ½ cup roasted vegetables): 517 calories; 50.7 g protein; 28.8 g total fat; 7.7 g saturated fat; 16.7 g carbohydrates; 1.5 g fiber; 250 mg sodium

PICTURED USING CHESTNUT FLOUR

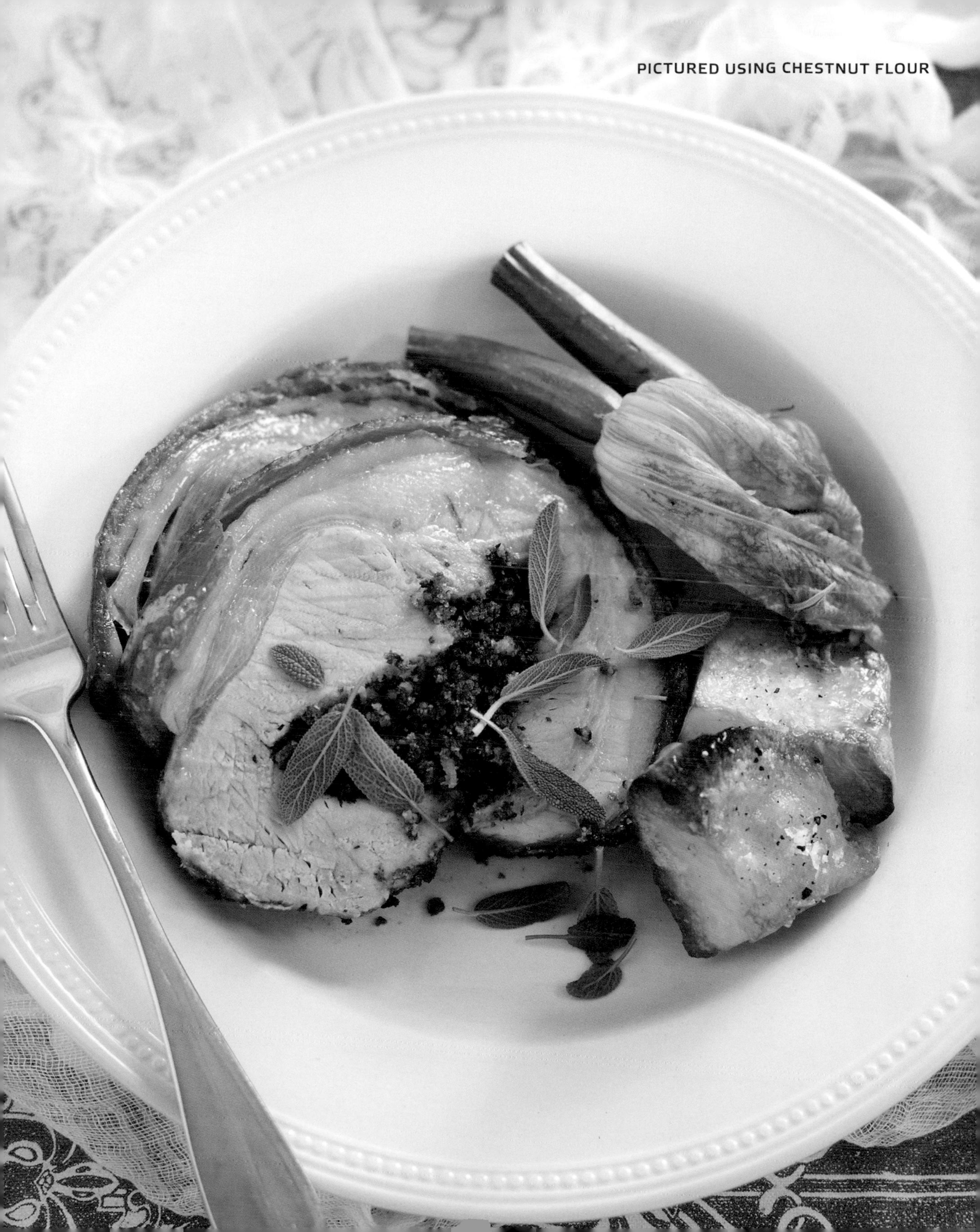

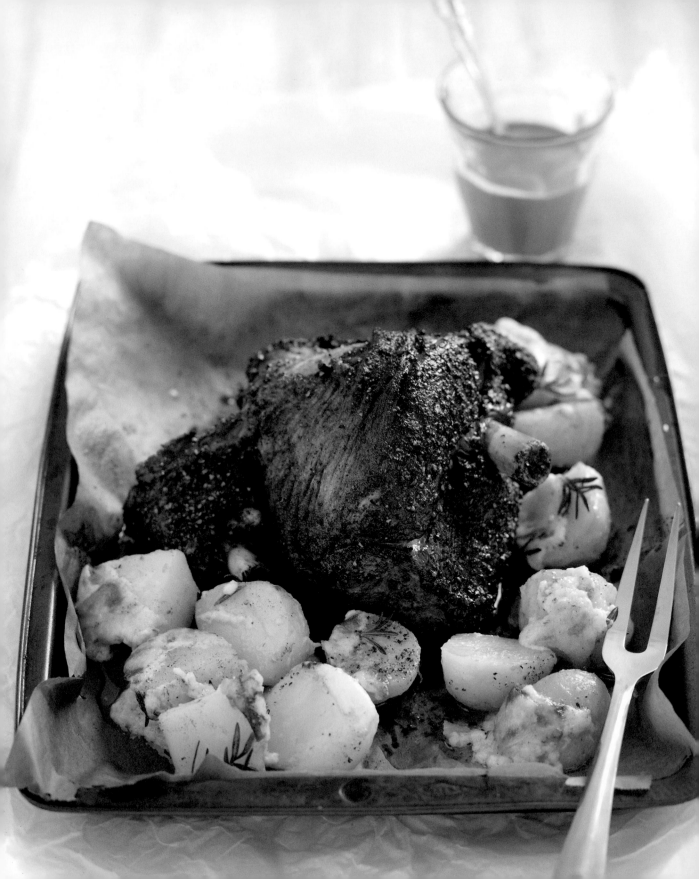

Peppered Lamb with Rosemary Cottage Potatoes

SERVES 8

The key to serving juicy, tender roast meat is to let it rest before you slice it. The fibers in the meat tighten during cooking, and the resting process allows them to relax. In this recipe, the lamb rests while the cottage potatoes are cooking.

1. Place the lamb in a roasting pan. Rub all over with the pepper, then cover with plastic wrap and refrigerate for 3 to 4 hours.

2. Preheat the oven to 400°F (200°C). Roast the lamb for 1 hour 20 minutes, until slightly pink in the middle and an instant-read thermometer inserted into the thickest part reaches 140°F (60°C) for medium, or until desired doneness. As soon as the lamb is out of the oven, remove it from the roasting pan and transfer to a plate. Cover with foil and let rest.

3. Meanwhile, place the potatoes in a large saucepan of cold water. Bring to a boil and cook for 10 to 12 minutes, until tender. Drain and cool, then peel and cut in half. Combine the potatoes and Cheddar in a large bowl and season with salt and pepper. Transfer the mixture to a medium baking dish.

4. Place the butter and rosemary in a small skillet over medium heat and stir until the butter is melted and lightly golden. Pour it over the potato mixture, followed by the milk. Bake the cottage potatoes for 20 to 25 minutes.

5. While the potatoes are baking, place the empty roasting pan on the stove over medium heat. Add the wine and cook for 5 minutes, or until the wine is reduced by half. Add the stock and bring to a boil. Reduce the heat and simmer, stirring regularly, for 5 minutes, or until the sauce starts to thicken. Remove the pan from the heat and stir in the sour cream until melted and well combined. Season with salt and pepper.

6. Carve the lamb and serve with the red wine sauce and cottage potatoes, with the steamed vegetables on the side.

PER SERVING: 638 calories; 63.5 g protein; 33.5 g total fat; 16.1 g saturated fat; 17.6 g carbohydrates; 2 g fiber; 427 mg sodium

3-pound (1.5 kg) leg of lamb

2 tablespoons freshly ground black pepper

ROSEMARY COTTAGE POTATOES

10 new potatoes

5 ounces (150 g) reduced-fat Cheddar, cubed (1 cup)

Salt and freshly ground black pepper

2 tablespoons (30 g) butter

2 tablespoons rosemary leaves

½ cup (125 ml) low-fat milk, lactose-free milk, or suitable plant-based milk

SAUCE

½ cup (125 ml) dry red wine, or onion-free beef stock (gluten-free if following a gluten-free diet)

1 cup (250 ml) onion-free beef stock (gluten-free if following a gluten-free diet)

3 tablespoons light sour cream

Salt and freshly ground black pepper

Steamed vegetables

Herbed Beef Meatballs with Creamy Mashed Potatoes

SERVES 6

This is a winter favorite for the whole family. The gravy tastes great with an added splash of red wine, but feel free to leave it out to suit younger palates.

1. To make the mashed potatoes, place the potatoes in a large saucepan and cover with cold water. Bring to a boil and cook for 15 minutes, or until tender when pierced with a fork. Drain and set aside for 5 minutes to cool slightly. Peel the potatoes and return to the pan. Add the remaining ingredients and mash with a potato masher until smooth. Cover and keep warm.

2. Meanwhile, combine the beef, bread crumbs, eggs, oregano, marjoram, and parsley in a large bowl. Season with salt and pepper. Roll the mixture into walnut-size balls.

3. Heat a little oil in a large heavy-bottomed skillet over medium heat. Add the meatballs and cook for 6 to 8 minutes, until browned and cooked through.

4. To make the gravy, combine the gravy powder, tomato paste, and red wine, if using, in a small bowl and stir well to form a paste. Slowly add 1 cup (250 ml) boiling water (or the amount called for in the gravy package instructions), stirring constantly to ensure there are no lumps and the gravy thickens evenly.

5. Divide the mashed potatoes among six plates and top with the meatballs. Spoon the gravy over the meatballs and garnish with the additional oregano.

PER SERVING: 276 calories; 13 g protein; 11.2 g total fat; 6.2 g saturated fat; 28.8 g carbohydrates; 2.7 g fiber; 530 mg sodium

CREAMY MASHED POTATOES

6 large russet potatoes

½ cup (125 ml) low-fat milk

3 tablespoons (45 g) butter

Pinch of salt

⅓ cup (40 g) coarsely grated reduced-fat Cheddar

Pinch of ground nutmeg

HERBED BEEF MEATBALLS

1¼ pounds (600 g) extra lean ground beef

½ cup (50 g) dried gluten-free bread crumbs

3 eggs, lightly beaten

2 tablespoons chopped oregano, plus additional leaves for garnish

2 tablespoons chopped marjoram

⅓ cup (10 g) chopped flat-leaf parsley

Salt and freshly ground black pepper

Canola oil

TOMATO GRAVY

3 tablespoons onion-free gravy powder (gluten-free if following a gluten-free diet)

2 tablespoons tomato paste

2 tablespoons dry red wine, optional

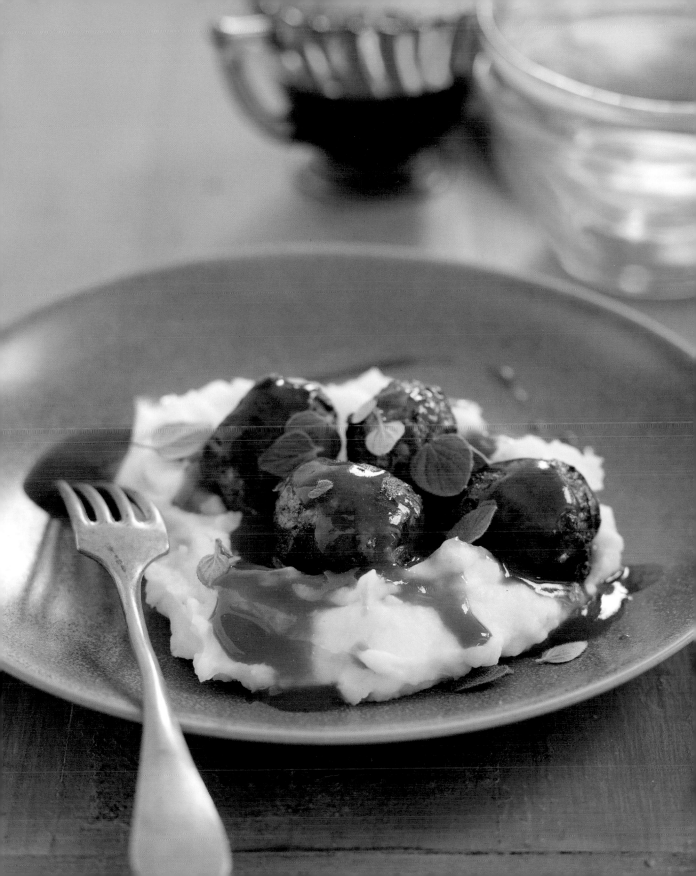

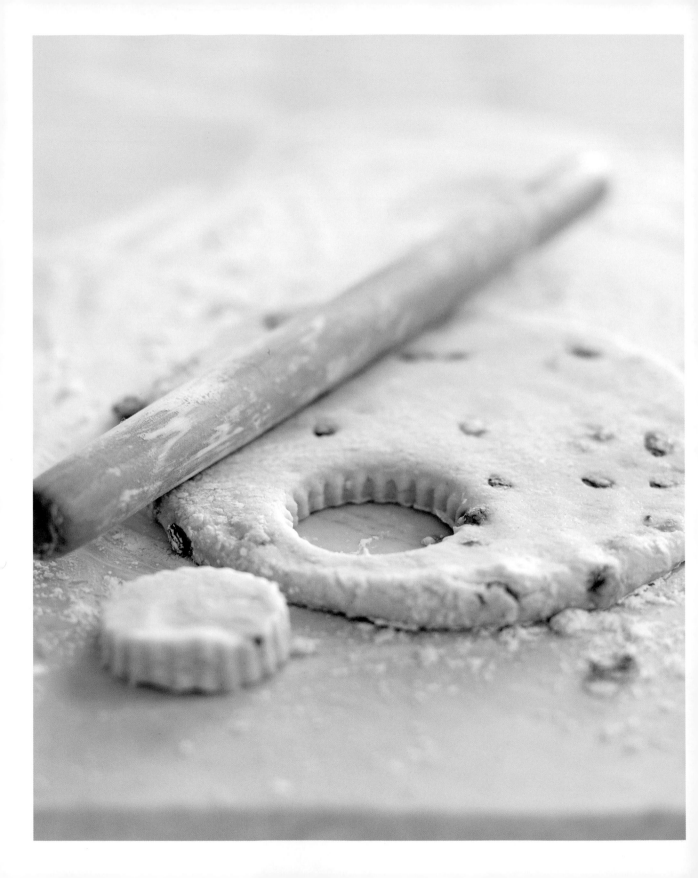

Breads and Baked Goods

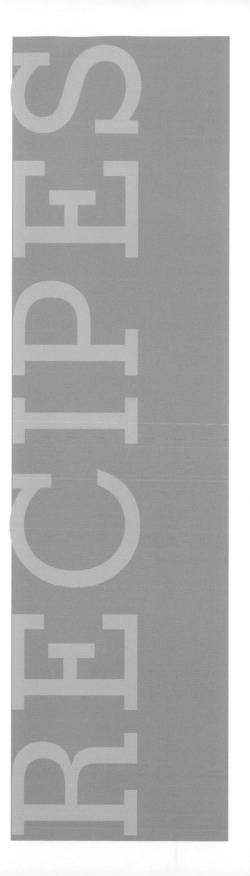

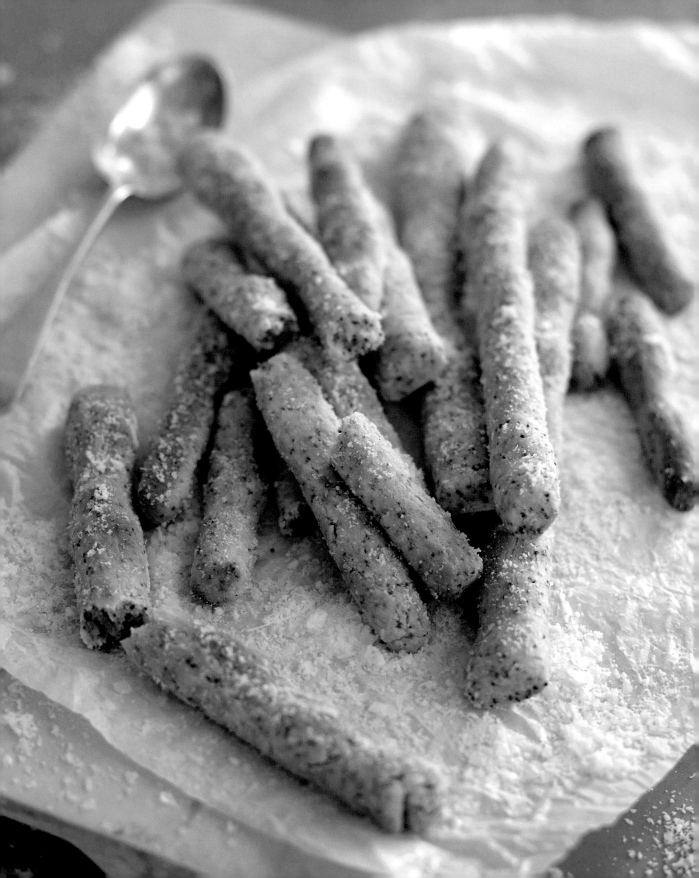

Poppy Seed, Pepper, and Cheese Sticks

MAKES 15 TO 30

For people with lactose intolerance, replace the cream cheese with soy cream cheese. The amount of soy flour used in this recipe is minimal, so it will suit most people following the low-FODMAP diet. Assess your individual tolerance.

One 8-ounce (250 g) package cream cheese

5 tablespoons (80 g) butter, softened

¾ cup (60 g) grated Parmesan

½ cup (65 g) fine rice flour

3 tablespoons cornstarch

3 tablespoons soy flour

1 teaspoon xanthan gum

2 tablespoons poppy seeds

1 teaspoon coarsely ground black pepper

Extra virgin olive oil

1. Place the cream cheese, butter, and ½ cup (40 g) Parmesan in a food processor and blend until smooth.

2. Sift the rice flour, cornstarch, soy flour, and xanthan gum three times into a large bowl (or mix with a whisk to ensure they are well combined). Stir in the poppy seeds and pepper. Add the cream cheese mixture and mix until just combined. Divide the dough into eight portions. Roll each portion on a flat surface into a 14-inch (35 cm) rope, then cut in half or into quarters to make sticks.

3. Line a large baking sheet with parchment paper. Place the sticks on the baking sheet and freeze for 20 minutes, or until firm.

4. Preheat the oven to 350°F (180°C). Line a second baking sheet with parchment paper and divide the frozen sticks between the two sheets, leaving space in between.

5. Bake the sticks for 12 to 15 minutes, until lightly golden brown and cooked through. Remove from the oven and allow them to cool on the baking sheets for 10 minutes before transferring to a clean baking sheet. Spray or brush with olive oil while still warm and roll in the remaining Parmesan. Store in an airtight container for up to 7 days.

PER SERVING (one thirtieth of recipe): 79 calories; 2.1 g protein; 6.2 g total fat; 3.6 g saturated fat; 4.0 g carbohydrates; 0.1 g fiber; 78 mg sodium

Two-Pepper Cornbread

SERVES 10

This savory loaf is made with coarse cornmeal, which adds a grainy texture to baked foods. It is delicious served freshly baked from the oven, but any leftovers will also toast up superbly.

1. Preheat the oven to 350°F (180°C). Lightly grease an 8 x 4-inch (20 x 9 cm) loaf pan and line with parchment paper.

2. Sift the rice flour, cornstarch, potato flour, baking powder, baking soda, and xanthan gum three times into a bowl (or mix with a whisk to ensure they are well combined). Stir in the corn-meal and salt.

3. Combine the eggs, milk, oil, chile peppers, bell pepper, and three quarters of the Parmesan and add to the flour mixture. Mix well to combine. Pour into the loaf pan and sprinkle with the re-maining cheese.

4. Bake for 35 to 45 minutes, until a toothpick inserted into the center comes out clean. Remove from the oven and allow to cool in the pan for 10 minutes before transferring to a wire rack to cool completely. Cut into slices and serve.

PER SERVING: 178 calories; 8.6 g protein; 6.1 g total fat; 3.2 g saturated fat; 21.8 g carbohydrates; 0.9 g fiber; 764 mg sodium

½ cup (65 g) fine rice flour

3 tablespoons cornstarch

3 tablespoons potato flour

2 teaspoons baking powder (gluten-free if following a gluten-free diet)

1 teaspoon baking soda

1 teaspoon xanthan gum

1 cup (125 g) coarse cornmeal

1 teaspoon salt

2 eggs, lightly beaten

1 cup (250 ml) low-fat milk, lactose-free milk, or suitable plant-based milk

1 teaspoon olive oil

2 small red chile peppers, seeded and finely chopped

½ red bell pepper, seeded and finely diced

1½ cups (120 g) grated Parmesan

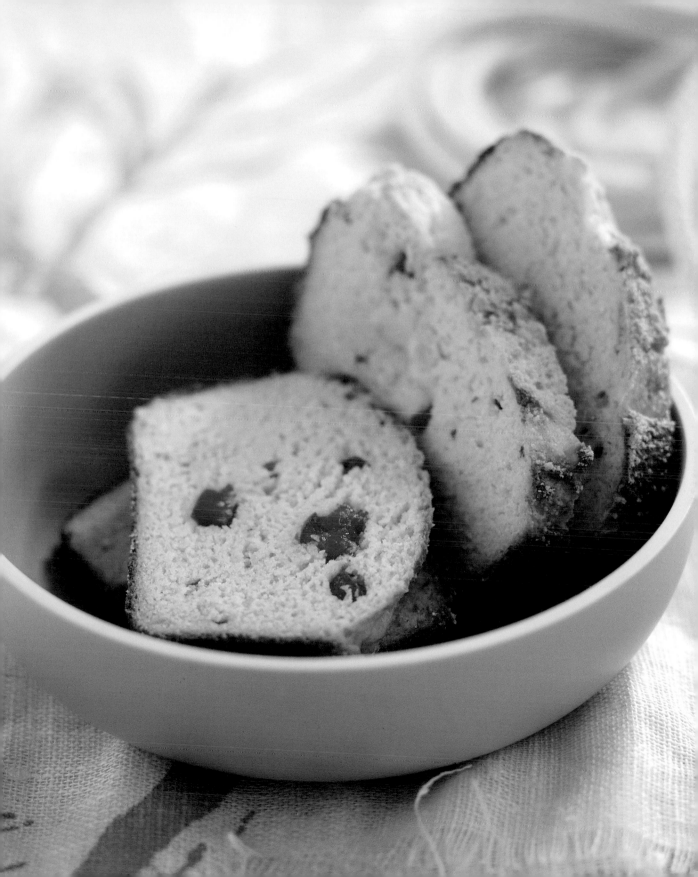

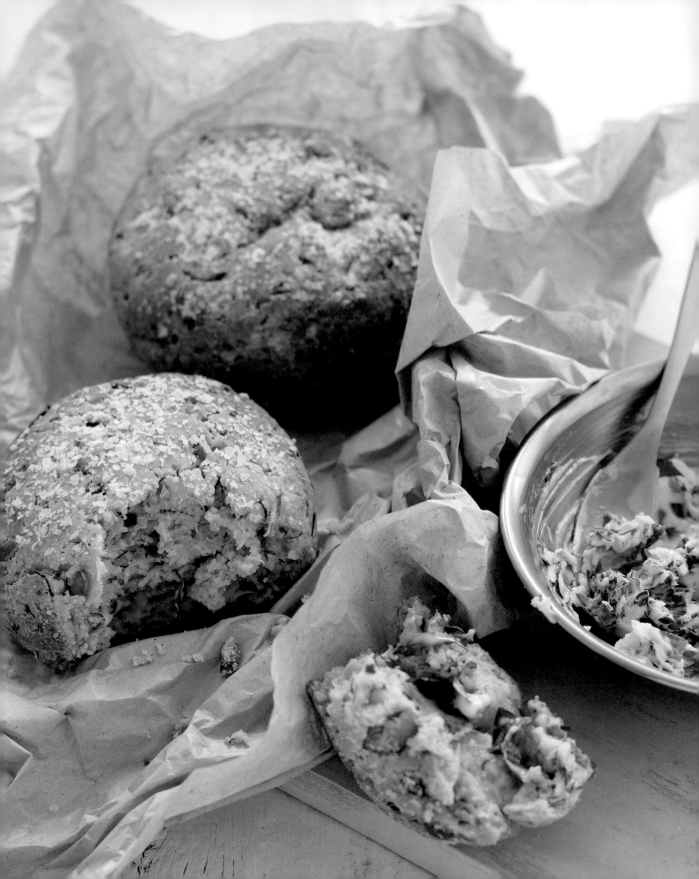

Zucchini and Pumpkin Seed Cornmeal Bread

SERVES 12

The grated zucchini keeps this loaf lovely and moist, while the pumpkin seeds give it a pleasing crunch. I like the parsley in the butter, but you can use other fresh herbs if preferred. The amount of soy flour used in this recipe is minimal, so it will suit most people following the low-FODMAP diet. Assess your individual tolerance—if necessary, you can replace the soy flour with tapioca flour.

1. Preheat the oven to 400°F (200°C) and line a baking sheet with parchment paper.

2. Sift the flours, baking powder, baking soda, and xanthan gum three times into a bowl (or mix with a whisk to ensure they are well combined). Stir in the cornmeal, zucchini, and pumpkin seeds. Make a well in the center and add the warmed milk and melted butter. Add the salt and pepper and mix well with a wooden spoon.

3. Gently bring the dough together with your hands to form a soft ball. Turn out onto a clean surface dusted with cornstarch and knead until smooth.

4. Divide the dough in half, form into two balls, and place on the baking sheet. Brush with a little oil and sprinkle with sea salt. Bake for 20 to 25 minutes, until golden brown and a toothpick inserted into the center comes out clean.

5. To make the parsley butter, mix together the butter and parsley in a bowl. Serve with the warm bread.

PER SERVING: 235 calories; 4.7 g protein; 10.6 g total fat; 4.9 g saturated fat; 29.6 g carbohydrates; 1.5 g fiber; 248 mg sodium

1 cup (130 g) fine rice flour

¾ cup (135 g) potato flour

½ cup (45 g) soy flour

2 teaspoons baking powder (gluten-free if following a gluten-free diet)

1 teaspoon baking soda

1 teaspoon xanthan gum

1 cup (125 g) cornmeal

1 large zucchini, grated and drained on paper towel

⅓ cup (65 g) raw or roasted pumpkin seeds

¾ cup plus 2 tablespoons (200 ml) warmed low-fat milk, lactose-free milk, or suitable plant-based milk

3 tablespoons (40 g) butter, melted

1 teaspoon salt

½ teaspoon freshly ground black pepper

Olive oil

Sea salt

PARSLEY BUTTER

4 tablespoons (55 g) butter

¼ cup (15 g) chopped flat-leaf parsley

Olive and Eggplant Focaccia

SERVES 6 TO 8

Things have come a long way in a few short years—these days, there is an abundance of gluten-free bread mixes available in supermarkets, health-food stores, and other retail outlets. They all vary in taste and texture, so you are sure to find one that suits you. Check that the mix does not include large amounts of FODMAP-containing flours (see page 78 for more information).

1. In a large shallow dish, mix together the oil, vinegar, parsley, oregano, and basil. Add the eggplant and turn to evenly coat, then let it marinate while you prepare the bread.

2. Preheat the oven to 350°F (180°C) and line a rimmed baking sheet with parchment paper. Make the gluten-free bread mix following the package directions and spoon onto the baking sheet. Using a spatula or the back of a spoon, spread out the mixture to cover the sheet (it should be about ¾-inch/2 cm thick).

3. Add a small amount of the eggplant marinade to a ridged grill pan or cast-iron skillet and heat over medium-high heat. Add the eggplant slices and cook, turning once, until lightly charred, 3 to 4 minutes.

4. Spread the pesto evenly over the bread dough using a spatula or the back of a metal spoon, dipping the spoon in water if required to keep it from sticking to the dough. Top with the olives, eggplant, and Parmesan, and season with salt and pepper. Bake for 25 to 35 minutes, until lightly browned. Remove from the oven and cool to room temperature on the baking sheet. Cut into pieces, sprinkle with the basil leaves, and serve warm.

PER SERVING (**one eighth of recipe**): 208 calories; 3.6 g protein; 12.6 g total fat; 2.9 g saturated fat; 20.4 g carbohydrates; 0.5 g fiber; 494 mg sodium

3 tablespoons garlic-infused olive oil

2 teaspoons balsamic vinegar

¼ teaspoon dried parsley

¼ teaspoon dried oregano

¼ teaspoon dried basil

½ small eggplant, cut into ½-inch (1 cm) slices

1 cup (280 g) gluten-free bread mix

3 tablespoons garlic-free basil pesto (gluten-free if following a gluten-free diet)

½ cup (75 g) sliced kalamata olives

½ cup (40 g) grated Parmesan

Salt and freshly ground black pepper

Small basil leaves

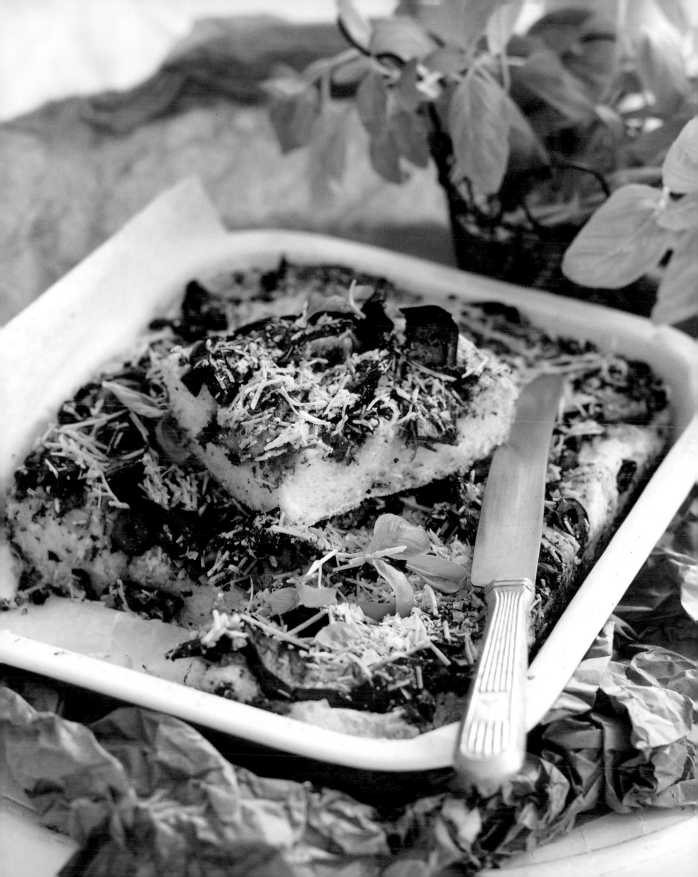

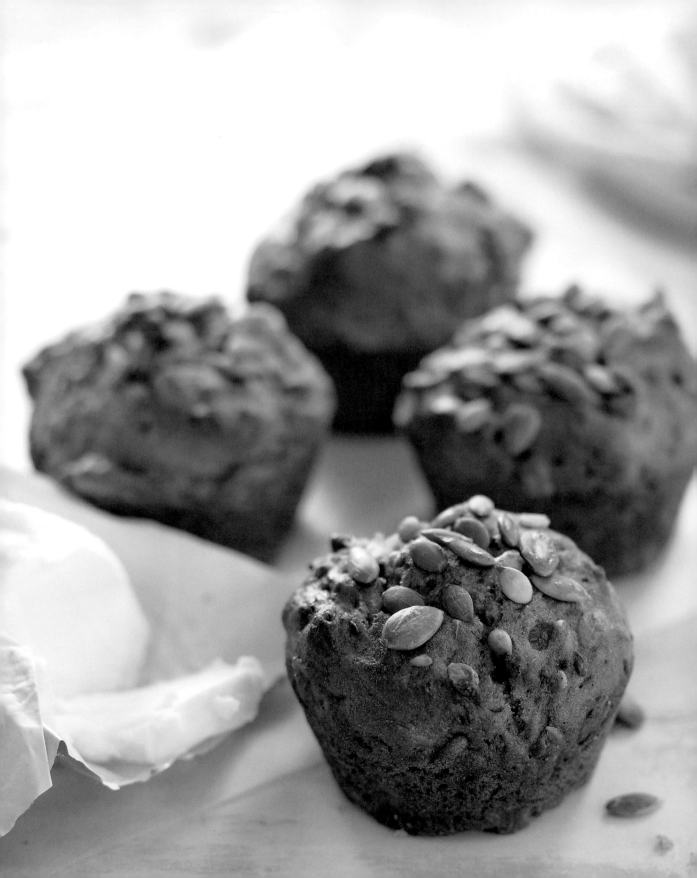

Chia Seed and Spice Muffins

MAKES 12

Chia seeds are packed with nutrition, making these muffins a wholesome snack, full of goodness and crunch. You could also spoon the mixture into a Texas muffin pan and enjoy these fragrant muffins for lunch. The amount of soy flour in this recipe is minimal so it will suit most people following the low-FODMAP diet. Assess your individual tolerance—if necessary, replace the soy flour with tapioca flour.

1. Preheat the oven to 350°F (170°C). Grease a 12-cup standard muffin pan.

2. Sift the brown rice flour, cornstarch, soy flour, baking powder, baking soda, pumpkin pie spice, cinnamon, and xanthan gum three times into a large bowl (or mix with a whisk to ensure they are well combined).

3. Place the eggs, oil, milk, chia seeds, sunflower seeds, ½ cup (100 g) of the pumpkin seeds, and the brown sugar in a medium bowl and mix with a wooden spoon until well combined. Pour into the sifted flours and mix well with a wooden spoon for 2 to 3 minutes.

4. Spoon the mixture into the muffin cups to two-thirds full and sprinkle the 2 tablespoons of pumpkin seeds evenly over the tops. Bake for 20 to 25 minutes, until firm to touch (a toothpick inserted into the center of the muffins should come out clean). Remove from the oven and allow to cool in the pan for 5 minutes before transferring to a wire rack to cool completely.

PER SERVING: 289 calories; 6.3 g protein; 17.8 g total fat; 2.5 g saturated fat; 25.8 g carbohydrates; 2 g fiber; 492 mg sodium

1 cup (140 g) brown rice flour

½ cup (75 g) cornstarch

½ cup (45 g) soy flour

2 teaspoons baking powder (gluten-free if following a gluten-free diet)

1 teaspoon baking soda

2 tablespoons pumpkin pie spice

1 tablespoon ground cinnamon

1 teaspoon xanthan gum

3 eggs

½ cup (125 ml) vegetable oil

½ cup (125 ml) low-fat milk, lactose-free milk, or suitable plant-based milk

⅓ cup (40 g) chia seeds

½ cup (40 g) hulled roasted sunflower seeds

⅓ cup (40 g) plus 2 tablespoons roasted pumpkin seeds

½ cup (110 g) brown sugar

Pineapple Muffins

MAKES 12

The crushed pineapple in these muffins adds a sweet flavor and moist texture that's hard to resist. Any muffins that don't disappear immediately can be frozen for another time.

1. Preheat the oven to 350°F (180°C). Line a 12-cup muffin pan with paper baking liners. Sift the rice flour, cornstarch, potato flour, baking soda, baking powder, and xanthan gum three times into a medium bowl (or mix with a whisk to ensure they are well combined). Add the sugar and mix until well combined.

2. Break the eggs into a bowl and whisk. Using a large spoon, stir in the melted butter, pineapple, and yogurt. Fold into the flour mixture.

3. Spoon the batter into the muffin liners. Bake for 15 to 20 minutes, until a toothpick inserted into the center of the muffins comes out clean. Remove from the oven and let cool in the pan for 5 minutes before transferring to a wire rack to cool completely.

4. Combine the confectioners' sugar with enough of the reserved pineapple liquid to form a smooth, spreadable icing. Drizzle over the cooled muffins and serve.

PER SERVING: 271 calories; 2.7 g protein; 7.4 g total fat; 4.5 g saturated fat; 49 g carbohydrates; 1.3 g fiber; 503 mg sodium

1 cup (130 g) fine rice flour

½ cup (75 g) cornstarch

½ cup (90 g) potato flour

1 teaspoon baking soda

2 teaspoons baking powder (gluten-free if following a gluten-free diet)

1 teaspoon xanthan gum

½ cup (110 g) superfine sugar

2 eggs

6 tablespoons (80 g) unsalted butter, melted

One 15.5-ounce (440 g) can crushed pineapple, drained (liquid reserved)

¾ cup (200 g) suitable low-fat vanilla yogurt (gluten-free if following a gluten-free diet)

1 cup (160 g) confectioners' sugar, sifted

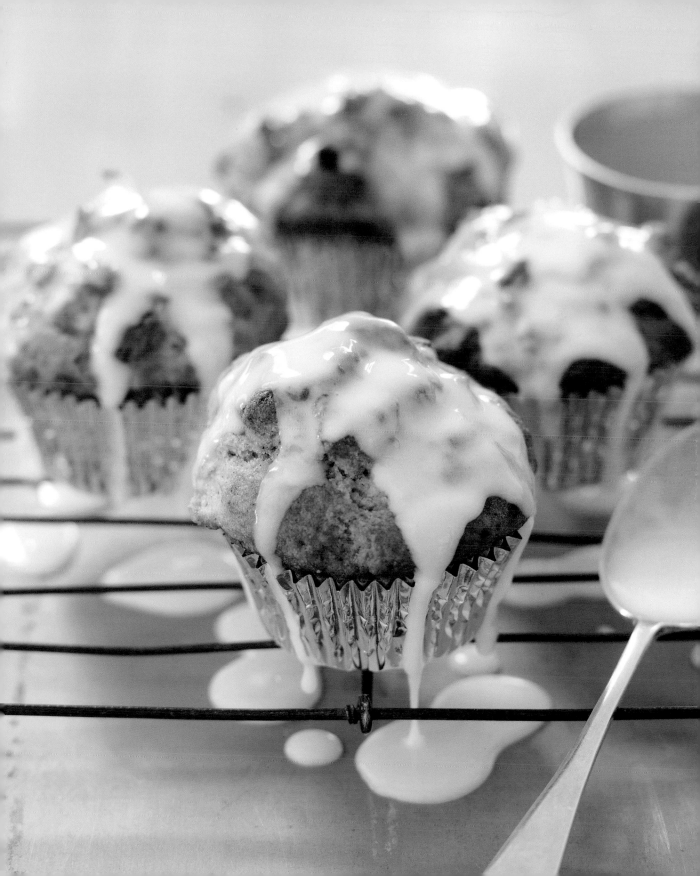

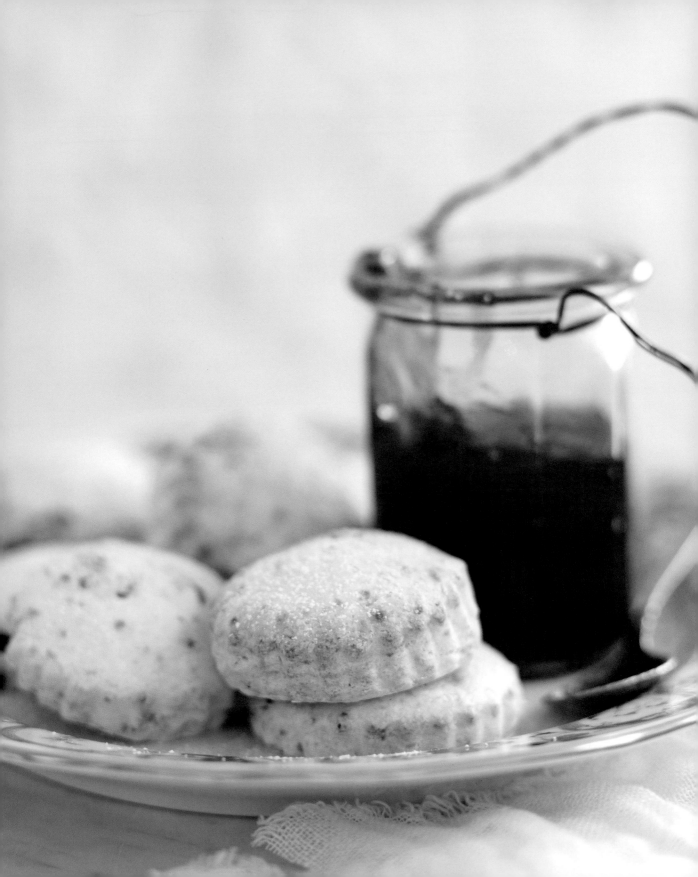

Breakfast Scones

MAKES 14

Here is a way for people following the low-FODMAP diet to enjoy this much-loved breakfast favorite. If you prefer your scones flavored, simply add ½ cup of blueberries or raspberries, or 2 tablespoons of roughly chopped nuts (all except pistachios or cashews). The amount of soy flour used in this recipe is minimal, so it will suit most people following the low-FODMAP diet. Assess your individual tolerance.

1. Preheat the oven to 400°F (200°C). Grease a baking sheet and dust with cornstarch.

2. Sift the cornstarch, tapioca flour, soy flour, xanthan gum, baking powder, and sugar three times into a large bowl (or mix with a whisk to ensure they are well combined). Cut in the butter until the mixture resembles fine bread crumbs.

3. Whisk 1 cup of the milk and the eggs in a bowl. Add to the flour mixture and stir until the dough begins to hold together. Gently bring the dough together with your hands and turn out onto a lightly floured surface. Knead gently four or five times until the dough is just smooth.

4. Roll out the dough to 1-inch (3 cm) thickness. Cut out the scones with a 2-inch (5 cm) biscuit or cookie cutter. Use a straight-down motion—if you twist the cutter, the scones will rise unevenly. Dipping the cutter in cornstarch before each cut also helps.

5. Place the scones on the baking sheet about ½ inch (1 cm) apart. Brush the tops with the remaining milk. Bake, rotating the sheet halfway through, for 15 to 18 minutes, until golden and cooked through. Remove the scones from the oven and wrap immediately in a clean kitchen towel (this gives them a soft crust). After 5 minutes, serve the scones with jam and whipped cream, if desired.

PER SERVING (not including jam or cream): 297 calories; 3.3 g protein; 11.6 g total fat; 6.4 g saturated fat; 45.5 g carbohydrates; 0.3 g fiber; 426 mg sodium

2 cups (300 g) cornstarch

2 cups (250 g) tapioca flour

1 cup (90 g) soy flour

2 teaspoons xanthan gum

1 tablespoon baking powder (gluten-free if following a gluten-free diet)

½ cup (110 g) superfine sugar

10 tablespoons (150 g) unsalted butter, at room temperature, cut into cubes

1¼ cups (300 ml) low-fat milk, plus 2 tablespoons (preferably cow's milk)

2 eggs

Jam, optional

Whipped cream, optional

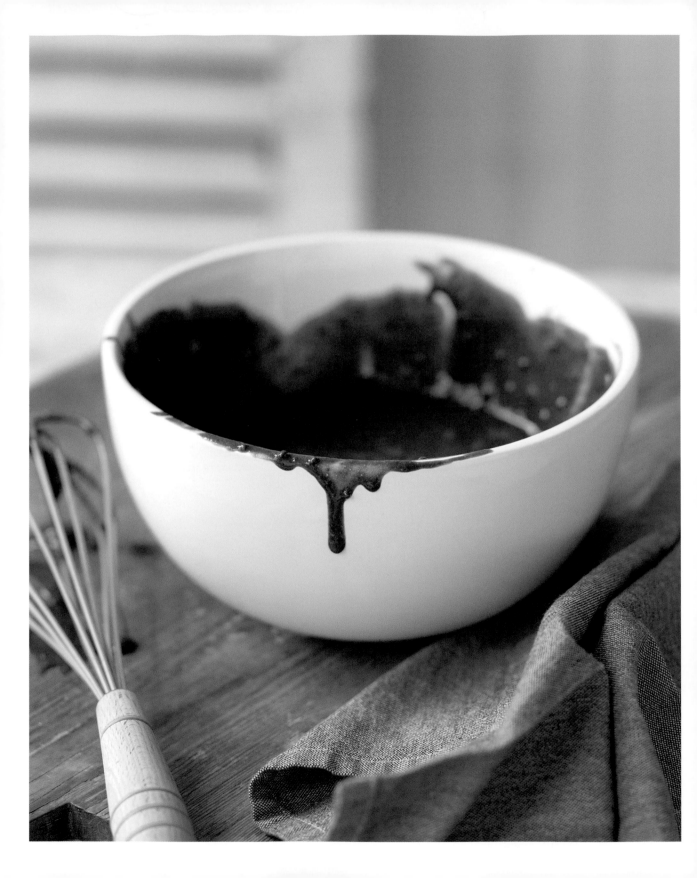

Cookies and Bars

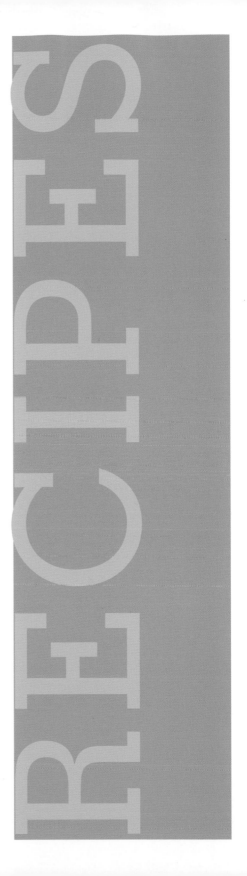

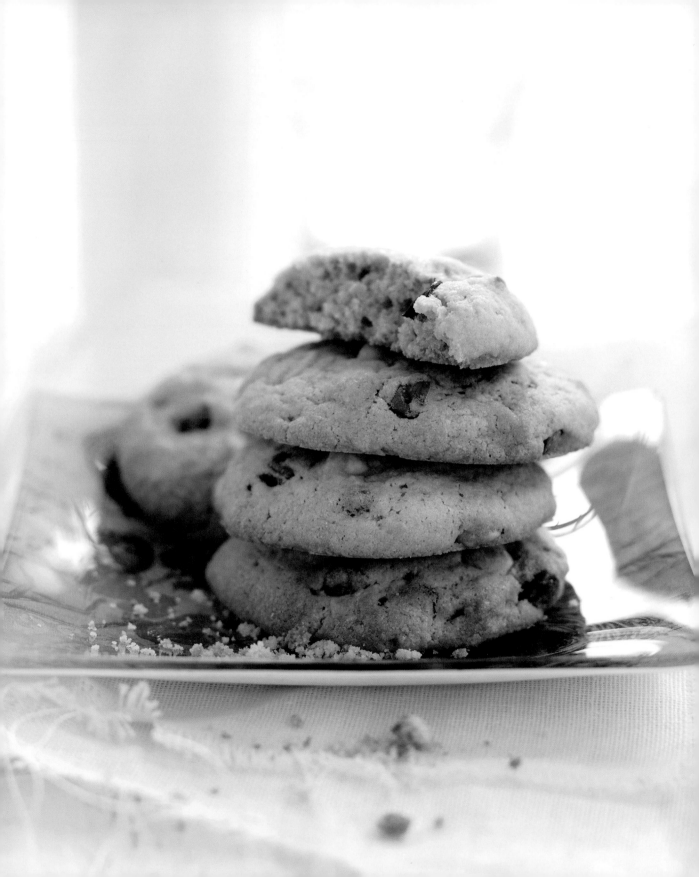

Chocolate Chip Cookies

MAKES 18

The amount of soy flour used here is minimal so these cookies should suit most people following the low-FODMAP diet. Assess your individual tolerance.

1. Preheat the oven to 350°F (180°C) and line two cookie sheets with parchment paper.

2. Beat the butter and brown sugar with an electric mixer until creamy. Add the eggs, one at a time, beating well between additions.

3. Sift the rice flour, cornstarch, soy flour, and xanthan gum three times into a bowl (or mix with a whisk to ensure they are well combined). Add to the butter mixture and stir until well combined. Mix in the chocolate chips, then gently bring the dough together with your hands. Roll the dough into golf-ball-size balls and place on the trays about 2 inches (5 cm) apart (to allow room for spreading). Flatten slightly with the back of a spoon.

4. Bake for 12 to 15 minutes, until golden. Cool on the cookie sheets for 10 minutes before transferring to a wire rack to cool completely.

PER SERVING: 236 calories; 2.7 g protein; 13.5 g total fat; 8.2 g saturated fat; 26.9 g carbohydrates; 0.3 g fiber; 25 mg sodium

14 tablespoons (200 g) unsalted butter, softened

¾ cup (165 g) brown sugar

2 eggs

1¼ cups (160 g) fine rice flour

⅓ cup (50 g) cornstarch

½ cup (45 g) soy flour

1 teaspoon xanthan gum

1 cup (180 g) chocolate chips (gluten-free if following a gluten-diet—white, milk, or dark, or use a mixture)

Lemon-Lime Bars

MAKES 20

This one is for those who love a sweet treat with a zesty twist. You'll want to start eating it as soon as it is baked, but try to resist the temptation—it behaves a lot better if you let it cool before slicing. The amount of soy flour used in this recipe is minimal so it will suit most people following the low-FODMAP diet. Assess your individual tolerance.

¾ cup (100 g) fine rice flour

½ cup (45 g) soy flour

½ cup (110 g) superfine sugar

2 teaspoons grated lemon zest

9 tablespoons (125 g) cold unsalted butter, roughly chopped

Confectioners' sugar

TOPPING

3 eggs

¾ cup (165 g) superfine sugar

3 tablespoons lemon juice

3 tablespoons ime juice

1 teaspoon grated lemon zest

3 tablespoons fine rice flour

1. Preheat the oven to 320°F (160°C). Grease and line an 8-inch (18 cm) square cake pan with parchment paper.

2. Place the flours, sugar, and lemon zest in a food processor and pulse until just combined. Add the butter, one piece at a time, and pulse until the mixture comes together in a ball. Remove and press into the pan. Bake for 10 minutes, or until lightly browned. Reduce the oven temperature to 300°F (150°C).

3. To make the topping, beat the eggs and sugar with an electric mixer until well combined but not thickened. Add the lemon and lime juices, lemon zest, and flours, and stir.

4. Pour the topping over the base and bake for 25 to 30 minutes, until golden. Allow to cool in the pan before cutting into slices. Dust with confectioners' sugar just before serving.

PER SERVING: 145 calories; 1.9 g protein; 6.5 g total fat; 3.7 g saturated fat; 20 g carbohydrates; 0.2 g fiber; 15 mg sodium

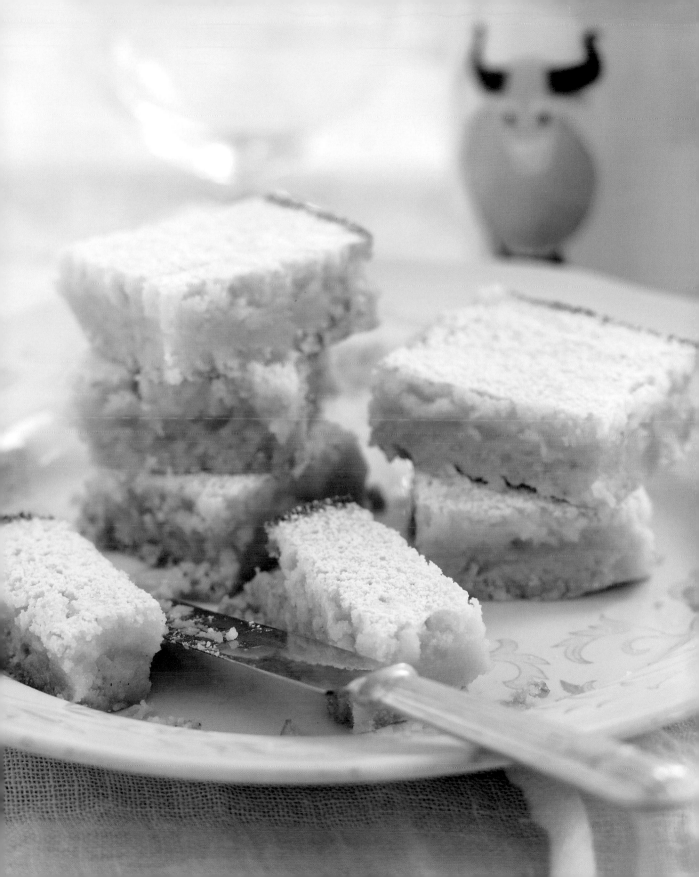

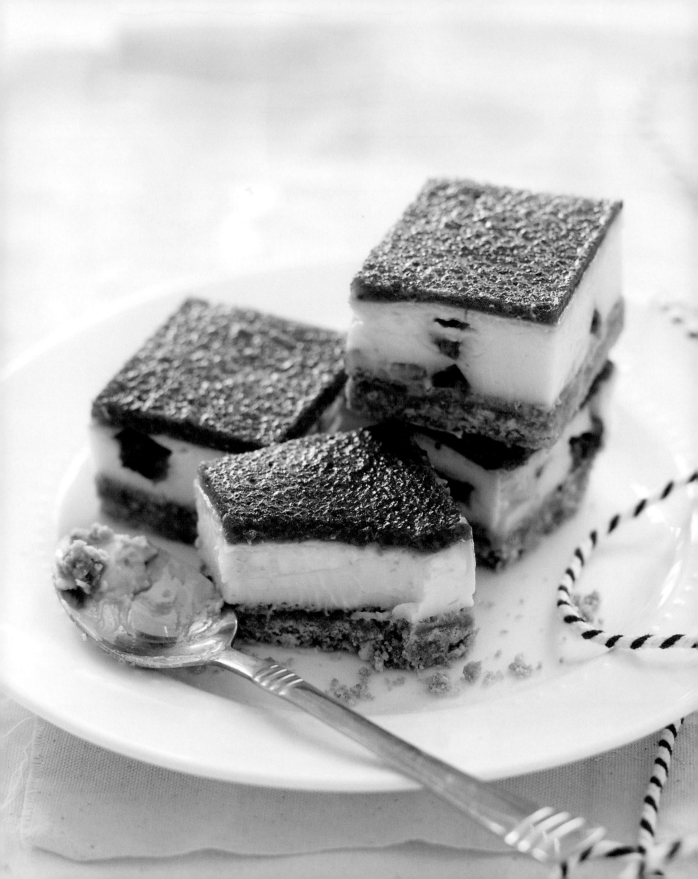

Strawberry Bars

MAKES 20

You could also use strawberry gelatin mix (made according to the package directions but using half the quantity of water) to top these delicious bars in place of the pureed strawberries. For people who are lactose intolerant, use lactose-free milk. Although a suitable plant-based milk may be substituted if absolutely necessary, this recipe works best with cow's milk.

1. Line a 9-inch (22 cm) square baking dish with parchment paper. Crush the cookies in a food processor.

2. Combine the butter and brown sugar in a medium saucepan and stir over medium-low heat until the butter has melted and the sugar has dissolved. Add the egg and stir until thickened. Add the cookie crumbs and mix well. Press into the bottom of the baking dish and set aside.

3. To make the filling, mix the cornstarch with a little milk to make a smooth paste. Gradually stir in the cream and remaining milk to combine. Add the sugar and vanilla, and cook gently over medium heat, stirring regularly with a wooden spoon, until the mixture is smooth and thick. Remove the pan from the heat and beat in the egg yolks. Set aside to cool for 5 to 10 minutes. Stir in the chopped strawberries. Pour the custard filling over the prepared crust. Refrigerate for 3 to 4 hours, until firm.

4. To make the topping, place the strawberries in a food processor and puree until smooth. Add 3 tablespoons of cold water to a small heatproof bowl and sprinkle the gelatin onto it while whisking with a fork. Set it aside for 5 minutes, or until it has begun to gel. Set the bowl in a larger bowl of boiling water and stir constantly until the gelatin has dissolved. Stir into the pureed strawberries.

5. Remove the dish from the fridge and pour the strawberry topping over the filling. Return to the fridge for 2 to 3 hours, until the topping is firm. Use a hot knife to cut into bars.

PER SERVING: 176 calories; 2.9 g protein; 10.2 g total fat; 6.2 g saturated fat; 19.1 g carbohydrates; 0.3 g fiber; 39 mg sodium

7 ounces (200 g) Simple Sweet Cookies (page 203), or other gluten-free vanilla cookies

6 tablespoons (80 g) unsalted butter

½ cup (110 g) brown sugar

1 egg, beaten

FILLING

½ cup (75 g) cornstarch

2 cups (500 ml) low-fat milk

¾ cup (185 ml) light whipping cream

⅓ cup (80 g) superfine sugar

2 teaspoons vanilla extract

2 egg yolks

4 ounces (100 g) strawberries, hulled and chopped (about ⅔ cup)

TOPPING

8 ounces (200 g) strawberries, hulled (about 1⅓ cups)

2 teaspoons unflavored gelatin

Brownies

MAKES 18 TO 20

These are so decadent, you had better stop at one . . . if you can!
Easy to prepare, and so very tempting, these rich brownies are
scrumptious with or without the addition of nuts.

1. Preheat the oven to 320°F (160°C). Line a 7 x 11-inch (29 x 19 cm)
baking pan with parchment paper and grease.

2. In a medium saucepan, melt the butter and dark chocolate
chunks over low heat. Stir until the mixture is smooth. Add the
brown sugar, stirring constantly until fully dissolved. Transfer the
mixture to a large bowl and let cool to room temperature.

3. Mix the fine rice flour, cornstarch, and xanthan gum together in a bowl with a whisk until well combined.

4. Stir the eggs into the chocolate mixture, one at a time. Add
the flours, chocolate chips, cream, and pecans. Spread the mixture in the prepared baking pan.

5. Bake for 20 minutes. Cover with foil and bake for another
20 to 25 minutes, until a toothpick inserted into the center comes
out clean. Remove from the oven and allow to cool in the pan to
room temperature, 30 to 40 minutes.

6. Transfer the pan to the refrigerator for 2 to 3 hours or overnight, until the brownies are firm. Remove from the refrigerator
and turn out onto a cutting board. Remove from the parchment
and cut into squares before serving.

PER SERVING (one twentieth of recipe): 298 calories; 2.9 g protein;
17.8 g total fat; 8.9 g saturated fat; 32.9 g carbohydrates; 0.7 g fiber; 27 mg sodium

10 tablespoons (150 g)
unsalted butter

8 ounces (250 g) dark
chocolate chunks

1½ cups (300 g) firmly packed
brown sugar

⅔ cup (130 g) fine rice flour

¼ cup (40 g) cornstarch

1 teaspoon xanthan gum

3 eggs, lightly beaten

½ cup (100 g) dark chocolate
chips (gluten-free if following a
gluten-free diet)

½ cup (125 ml) light whipping
cream

1 cup (100 g) chopped pecans

Cakes and Tarts

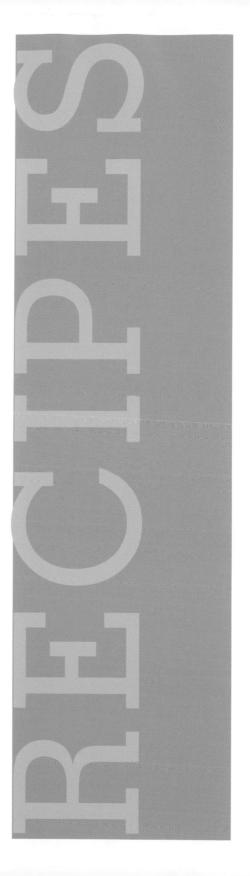

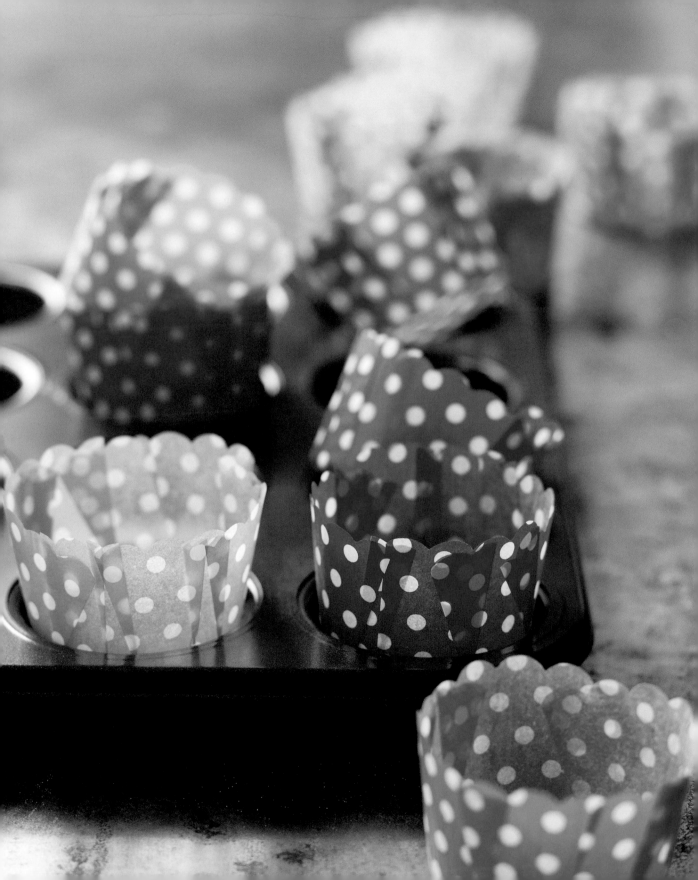

Basic Chocolate Cake

SERVES 10 TO 12

This is chocolate cake that everyone in the family will enjoy—I know this from experience! People following a lactose-free diet should choose lactose-free milk and yogurt. If you have a party coming up, you can make festive cupcakes using this recipe. Line a 12-cup muffin pan with muffin liners, fill each three-quarters full, and bake for 15 to 20 minutes, then top with whipped cream or your favorite frosting.

1. Preheat the oven to 350°F (170°C) and grease a 9-inch (23 cm) springform pan.

2. Sift the rice flour, cornstarch, potato flour, cocoa powder, baking powder, baking soda, and xanthan gum three times into a large bowl (or mix with a whisk so they are well combined).

3. Whisk the eggs and sugar until thick and foamy. Add the melted butter, yogurt, and milk, and stir until well combined. Pour the mixture into the sifted flours and beat with an electric mixer for 2 to 3 minutes.

4. Pour the batter into the pan and bake for 45 to 55 minutes, until firm to the touch (a toothpick inserted into the center should come out clean). Cover with foil halfway through baking to prevent overbrowning. Remove from the oven and allow the cake to cool in the pan for 5 minutes before transferring to a wire rack to cool completely.

5. Dust with confectioners' sugar and serve with a dollop of whipped cream.

PER SERVING (one twelfth of recipe, not including confectioners' sugar or whipped cream): 287 calories; 4.3 g protein; 5.7 g total fat; 3.3 g saturated fat; 54.9 g carbohydrates; 2.3 g fiber; 503 mg sodium

1 cup plus 2 tablespoons (170 g) fine rice flour

½ cup (75 g) cornstarch

½ cup (90 g) potato flour

⅔ cup (70 g) cocoa powder

2 teaspoons baking powder (gluten-free if following a gluten-free diet)

1 teaspoon baking soda

1 teaspoon xanthan gum

2 eggs

1½ cups (330 g) sugar

3 tablespoons (50 g) unsalted butter, melted

¾ cup (200 g) vanilla yogurt (gluten-free if following a gluten-free diet)

⅔ cup (170 ml) low-fat milk, lactose-free milk, or suitable plant-based milk

Confectioners' sugar

Whipped cream

Mocha Mud Cake

SERVES 12 TO 14

The secret of this delicious chocolate cake is the subtle coffee flavor in the background. If you love a stronger coffee hit, use the very strongest coffee you can, to enhance the impact of this feature ingredient. There are no leaveners in this recipe—it is a low, nonrising cake, the way a good mud cake should be! Rich and dense, a small serving is all you need.

1. Preheat the oven to 320°F (160°C). Grease and line an 8-inch (20 cm) round cake pan.

2. Place the coffee, chocolate chips, butter, vanilla, and cocoa powder in a medium glass bowl. Set over a saucepan of simmering water (make sure the bottom of the bowl does not touch the water) and stir until the chocolate has melted and is well combined.

3. Place the sugar and eggs in a large bowl, and beat with an electric mixer on high for 3 to 5 minutes, until light, fluffy, and doubled in volume. With a spoon, gradually fold in the chocolate mixture, stirring gently to combine.

4. Sift the rice flour, potato flour, cornstarch, and xanthan gum three times into a large bowl (or mix with a whisk to ensure they are well combined). Gradually fold into the chocolate mixture.

5. Pour the batter into the pan and bake for 50 to 60 minutes, until a toothpick inserted into the center comes out clean. Remove from the oven and allow to cool in the pan for 15 minutes before transferring to a wire rack to cool completely. Dust with extra cocoa powder, if desired, and serve.

PER SERVING (one fourteenth of recipe): 289 calories; 2.9 g protein; 15.9 g total fat; 9.8 g saturated fat; 34.1 g carbohydrates; 1.1 g fiber; 109 mg sodium

3 tablespoons strong coffee

7 ounces (200 g) dark chocolate chips (gluten-free if following a gluten-free diet)

12 tablespoons (180 g) butter, chopped

1 teaspoon vanilla extract

⅓ cup (35 g) cocoa powder, plus additional for dusting, optional

1 cup (220 g) superfine sugar

3 eggs

½ cup (65 g) fine rice flour

¼ cup (45 g) potato flour

¼ cup (40 g) cornstarch

1 teaspoon xanthan gum

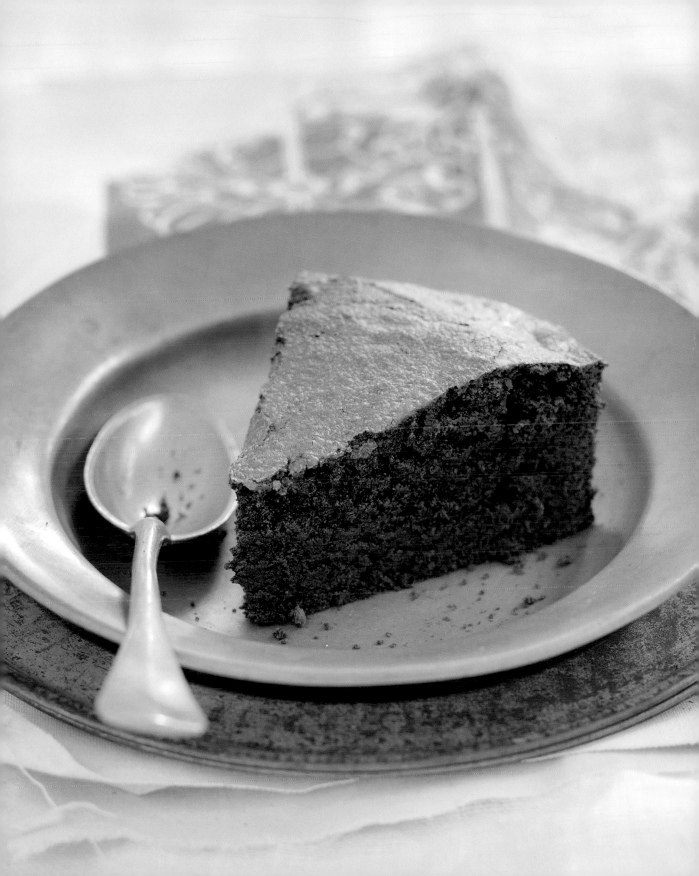

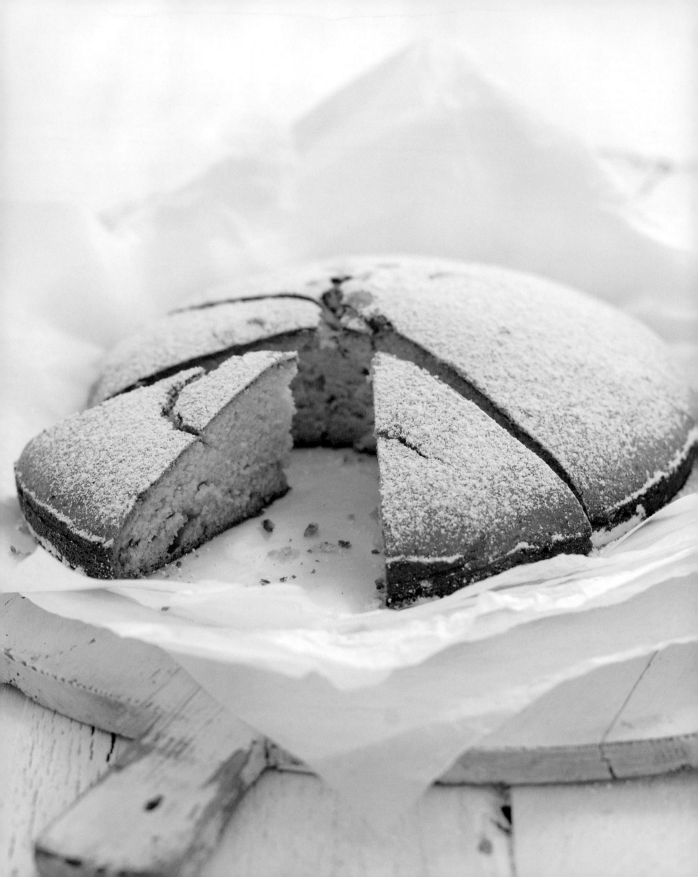

Vanilla Cake

SERVES 10 TO 12

It is preferable to use fine rice flour for baking, as regular rice flour can give a grainy mouthfeel. Fine rice flour is available from Asian grocers and many larger supermarkets. For people with lactose intolerance, use lactose-free yogurt and milk.

1. Preheat the oven to 350°F (170°C) and grease a 9-inch (23 cm) springform pan.

2. Sift the rice flour, cornstarch, potato flour, baking powder, baking soda, and xanthan gum three times into a large bowl (or mix with a whisk to ensure they are well combined).

3. Whisk together the eggs, sugar, and vanilla until thick and foamy. Add the melted butter, yogurt, and milk, and stir until well combined. Pour into the sifted flours and beat with an electric mixer for 2 to 3 minutes.

4. Pour the batter into the pan and bake for 30 to 35 minutes, until firm to touch (a toothpick inserted into the center should come out clean). Remove from the oven and allow the cake to cool in the pan for 5 minutes before transferring to a wire rack to cool completely. Dust with confectioners' sugar and serve.

PER SERVING (one twelfth of recipe, not including confectioners' sugar): 218 calories; 3g protein; 4.7 g total fat, 2.7 g saturated fat; 41.6 g carbohydrates; 0.6 g fiber; 513 mg sodium

1 cup (130 g) fine rice flour

½ cup (75 g) cornstarch

½ cup (90 g) potato flour

2 teaspoons baking powder (gluten-free if following a gluten-free diet)

1 teaspoon baking soda

1 teaspoon xanthan gum

2 eggs

1 cup (220 g) sugar

3½ teaspoons vanilla extract

3 tablespoons (50 g) butter, melted

¾ cup (200 g) vanilla yogurt (gluten-free if following a gluten-free diet)

⅔ cup (170 ml) low-fat milk, lactose-free milk, or suitable plant-based milk

Confectioners' sugar

Carrot and Pecan Cake

SERVES 12

This moist, flavorful cake needs no adornment and is perfect for an afternoon or after-dinner snack. Tapioca flour can be purchased at Asian grocers and in the Asian section of larger supermarkets. You could add chopped crystallized ginger, a small handful of dried cranberries, or 2 tablespoons of pumpkin pie spice as variations on this great basic recipe.

1. Preheat the oven to 350°F (170°C). Grease an 8 x 4-inch (20 x 9 cm) loaf pan and line with parchment paper.

2. Sift the rice flour, cornstarch, tapioca flour, cinnamon, baking soda, baking powder, and xanthan gum three times into a medium bowl (or mix with a whisk to ensure they are well combined). Stir in the brown sugar and chopped pecans. Add the grated carrots, oil, eggs, and milk, and mix well with a wooden spoon.

3. Spoon the batter into the pan and smooth the surface. Bake for about 1 hour, or until golden brown (a toothpick inserted into the center should come out clean). Cover with foil halfway through baking to prevent overbrowning. Remove from the oven and allow to cool in the pan for 10 minutes before transferring to a wire rack to cool completely.

PER SERVING: 310 calories; 3.5 g protein; 16.5 g total fat; 2.1 g saturated fat; 38 g carbohydrates; 1.1 g fiber; 488 mg sodium

1 cup (130 g) fine rice flour

½ cup (75 g) cornstarch

½ cup (65 g) tapioca flour

2 teaspoons ground cinnamon

1 teaspoon baking soda

2 teaspoons baking powder (gluten-free if following a gluten-free diet)

1 teaspoon xanthan gum

1 cup (220 g) brown sugar

¾ cup (90 g) chopped pecans

2 small carrots, peeled and grated

½ cup (125 ml) vegetable oil

3 eggs, lightly beaten

½ cup (125 ml) low-fat milk, lactose-free milk, or suitable plant-based milk

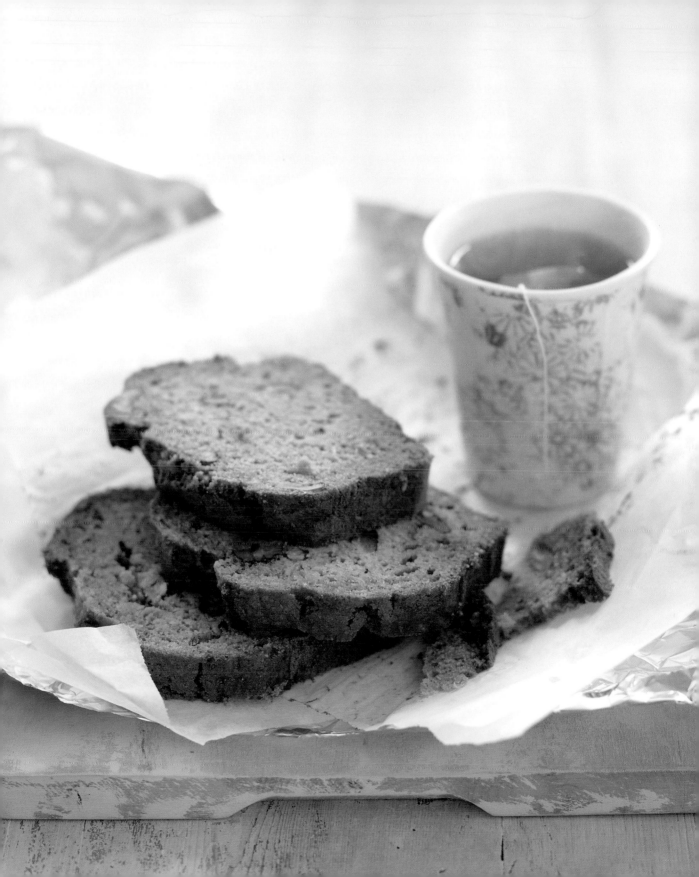

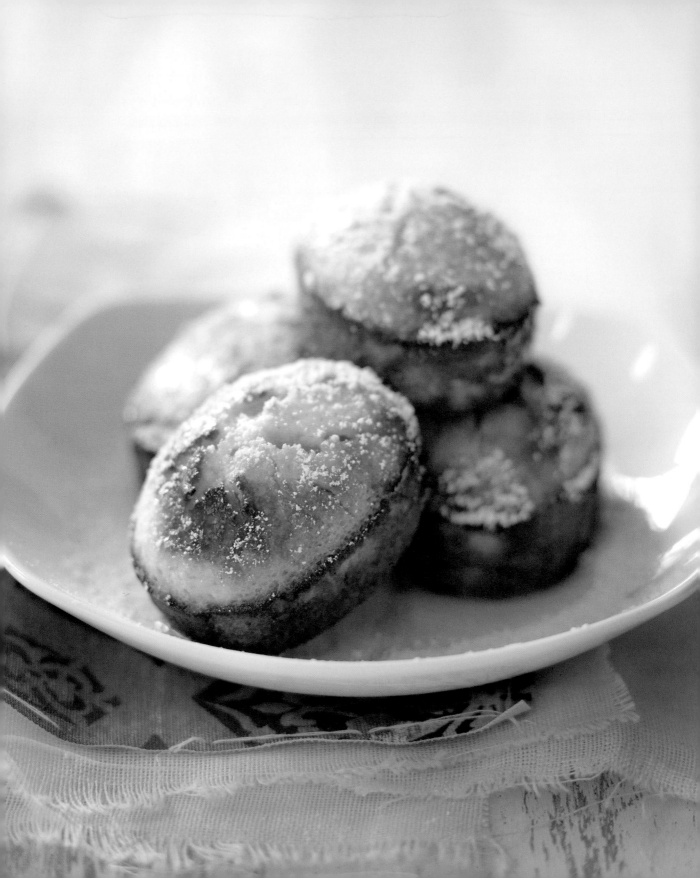

Lemon Friands
(Mini Almond Cakes)

MAKES 12

These miniature almond cakes are a delight on their own or simply dusted with confectioners' sugar. If you want to dress them up, the lemon glaze makes a delicious addition.

1. Preheat the oven to 350°F (180°C). Lightly grease a 12-cup muffin pan, or 12 friand pans or petite loaf pans. Melt the butter in a small saucepan over low heat. Cook for 3 to 4 minutes, until you start to see flecks of brown appear. Remove from the heat.

2. Sift the confectioners' sugar, cornstarch, and rice flour three times into a bowl (or mix with a whisk to ensure they are well combined). Stir in the ground almonds and lemon zest. Add the egg whites, lemon juice, vanilla, and melted butter, and mix well.

3. Spoon the mixture into the cups to two-thirds full. Bake for 12 to 15 minutes, until light golden and firm to touch. Remove from the oven and allow to cool in the pan for 5 minutes before transferring to a wire rack to cool completely.

4. Meanwhile, to make the glaze, place the lemon juice and zest, sugar, butter, and cornstarch with 2 tablespoons hot water in a small heavy-bottomed saucepan over low heat and cook, stirring constantly, for 10 minutes, or until thickened. Remove from the heat and cool to room temperature.

5. Drizzle the lemon glaze over the cakes and dust with confectioners' sugar.

PER SERVING: 342 calories; 4.2 g protein; 19.5 g total fat; 8.6 g saturated fat; 39.3 g carbohydrates; 1.2 g fiber; 26 mg sodium

10 tablespoons (140 g) unsalted butter

2 cups (320 g) confectioners' sugar, plus additional for dusting

3 tablespoons cornstarch

3 tablespoons rice flour

1¼ cups (140 g) ground almonds

Finely grated zest of 1 lemon

5 egg whites, lightly whisked

2 tablespoons lemon juice

1 teaspoon vanilla extract

LEMON GLAZE

Juice of 1 lemon

1 teaspoon finely grated lemon zest

⅓ cup (75 g) superfine sugar

3 tablespoons (40 g) unsalted butter

½ teaspoon cornstarch

Moist Banana Cake

SERVES 12

This fragrant cake is delicious served warm. For an extra treat, spread it with a little butter, which will melt beautifully into the moist cake.

1. Preheat the oven to 350°F (170°C) and grease an 8 x 4-inch (20 x 9 cm) loaf pan.

2. Sift the rice flour, cornstarch, potato flour, baking soda, baking powder, xanthan gum, and spices three times into a large bowl (or mix with a whisk to ensure they are well combined).

3. Mix together the oil, yogurt, and eggs in a medium bowl. Stir in the bananas and brown sugar. Add to the dry ingredients and beat with an electric mixer for 2 to 3 minutes.

4. Pour the batter into the pan and bake for 45 to 55 minutes, until golden brown (a toothpick inserted into the center should come out clean). Cover with foil halfway through baking to prevent overbrowning. Remove from the oven and allow to cool in the pan for 5 minutes before transferring to a wire rack to cool completely. Serve as is or spread with butter.

PER SERVING: 225 calories; 2.7 g protein; 4.7 g total fat; 0.6 g saturated fat; 43.4 g carbohydrates; 1.1 g fiber; 485 mg sodium

1 cup (130 g) fine rice flour

½ cup (75 g) cornstarch

½ cup (90 g) potato flour

1 teaspoon baking soda

2 teaspoons baking powder (gluten-free if following a gluten-free diet)

1 teaspoon xanthan gum

2 teaspoons pumpkin pie spice

1 teaspoon ground cinnamon

3 tablespoons canola oil

¾ cup (200 g) suitable low-fat vanilla yogurt (gluten-free if following a gluten-free diet)

2 eggs

2 ripe bananas, mashed

1 cup (220 g) brown sugar

Butter, optional

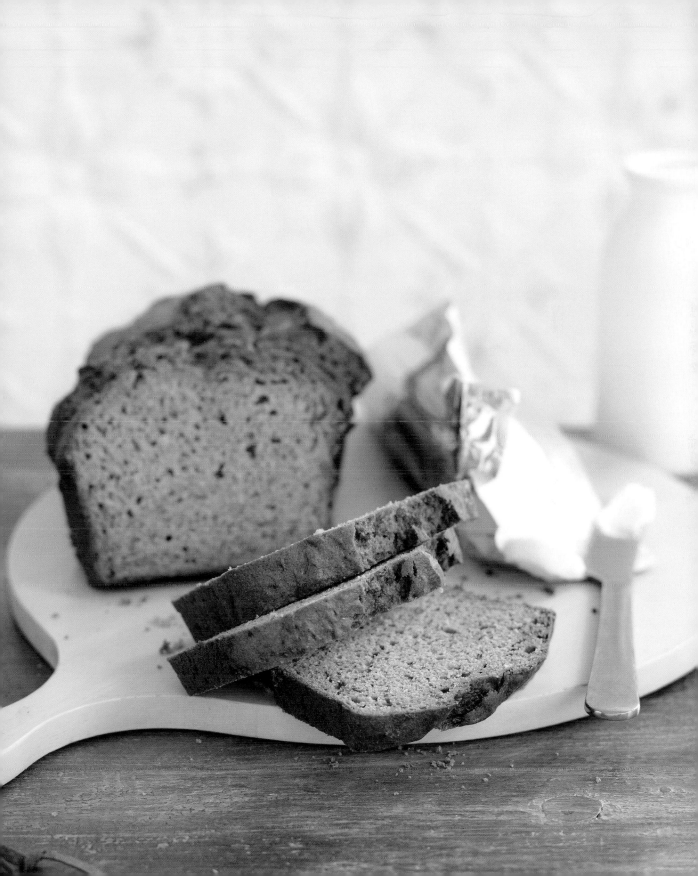

PICTURED USING CHESTNUT FLOUR

Sweet Almond Cake

SERVES 12

This is a lovely moist cake with a delicate sweetness. You may serve it with fresh strawberries or blueberries, and it also tastes wickedly good with whipped cream. If you can find chestnut flour, it's a handy replacement for those allergic to nuts, as chestnuts are not actually nuts at all!

1. Preheat the oven to 350°F (180°C). Grease a 9-inch (24-cm) springform pan and dust with cornstarch.

2. Sift the rice flour, cornstarch, baking powder, baking soda, and xanthan gum three times into a bowl (or mix with a whisk to ensure they are well combined).

3. Place the egg yolks and ½ cup (110 g) of the sugar in a medium bowl and beat with an electric mixer for 5 to 6 minutes, until thick, creamy, and doubled in volume. With a spoon, gently beat in the yogurt, oil, and vanilla. Fold in the sifted flours and almond flour.

4. Beat the egg whites in a clean bowl for 5 minutes, or until soft peaks form. Add the remaining ½ cup (110 g) of sugar and beat until stiff peaks form. Gently fold half of the egg whites into the almond mixture, then fold in the remaining egg whites.

5. Pour the batter into the pan. Bake for 1 hour 20 minutes, or until golden brown (a toothpick inserted into the center should come out clean). Cover with foil halfway through baking to prevent overbrowning. Remove from the oven and allow to cool in the pan for 10 minutes before transferring to a wire rack to cool completely. Dust with confectioners' sugar and serve with whipped cream, if desired.

PER SERVING (not including confectioners' sugar or whipped cream): 317 calories; 6.7 g protein; 18.8 g total fat; 1.9 g saturated fat; 31.3 g carbohydrates; 1.1 g fiber; 503 mg sodium

½ cup (65 g) fine rice flour

½ cup (75 g) cornstarch

2 teaspoons baking powder (gluten-free if following a gluten-free diet)

1 teaspoon baking soda

1 teaspoon xanthan gum

6 eggs, separated

1 cup (220 g) superfine sugar

¾ cup (200 g) suitable low-fat vanilla yogurt (gluten-free if following a gluten-free diet)

½ cup (125 ml) canola oil

1 teaspoon vanilla extract

1 cup (145 g) almond flour, preferably blanched, or chestnut flour

Confectioners' sugar

Whipped cream, optional

New York Cheesecake

SERVES 16

It is hard to resist going back for seconds (and thirds) of this classic dessert. It's gorgeous on its own but can also be dressed up with whipped cream and fresh raspberries. If you are lactose intolerant, only try a few bites.

1. Grease a 9-inch (22 cm) springform pan and line with parchment paper. Crush the cookies in a food processor and add the melted butter. Pulse to combine. Press onto the bottom and sides of the pan. Cover with plastic wrap and refrigerate for 1 hour.

2. Preheat the oven to 320°F (160°C).

3. Beat the cream cheese, sugar, vanilla, lemon zest, and cornstarch with an electric mixer until well combined. Add the eggs, one at a time, beating well between additions. Pour in the cream and mix until just combined.

4. Pour the cream cheese mixture over the cookie base. Bake for 1¼ to 1½ hours, until just set in the center (it should be firm when gently shaken). Turn the oven off and leave the cheesecake to cool in the oven with the door ajar for about 2 hours. Place in the refrigerator to cool completely. Decorate with the raspberries and dust with confectioners' sugar before serving.

PER SERVING (including raspberries): 392 calories; 6.7 g protein; 31.2 g total fat; 19.5 g saturated fat; 22.9 g carbohydrates; 0.5 g fiber; 203 mg sodium

7 ounces (200 g) Simple Sweet Cookies (see page 203), or other gluten-free vanilla cookies

7 tablespoons unsalted butter, melted

Three 8-ounce packages (750 g) cream cheese, at room temperature

1 cup (220 g) superfine sugar

2 teaspoons vanilla extract

2 teaspoons finely grated lemon zest

2 tablespoons cornstarch

4 eggs

1¼ cups (300 ml) light whipping cream

¾ cup (100 g) fresh raspberries

Confectioners' sugar

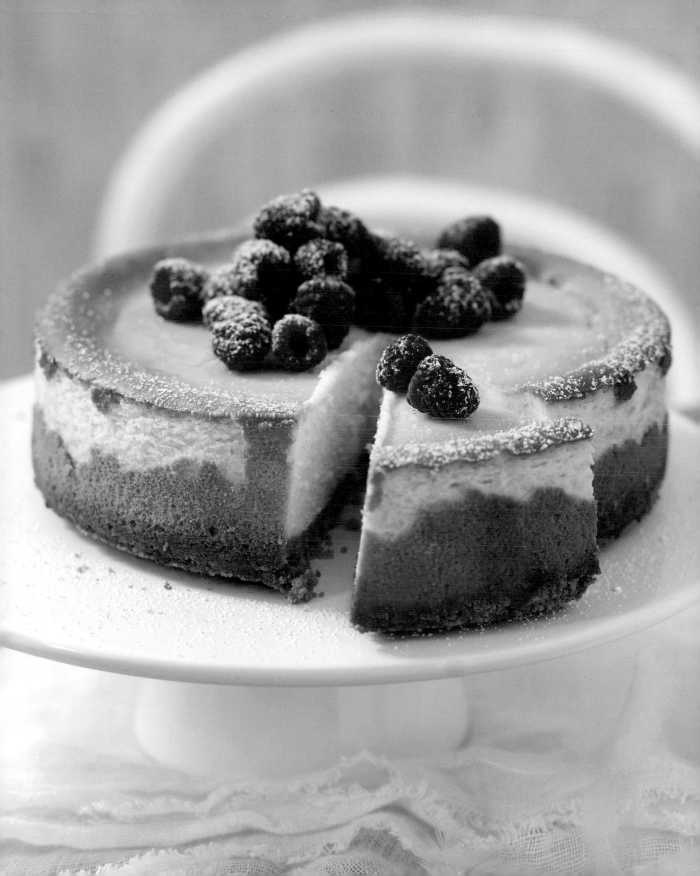

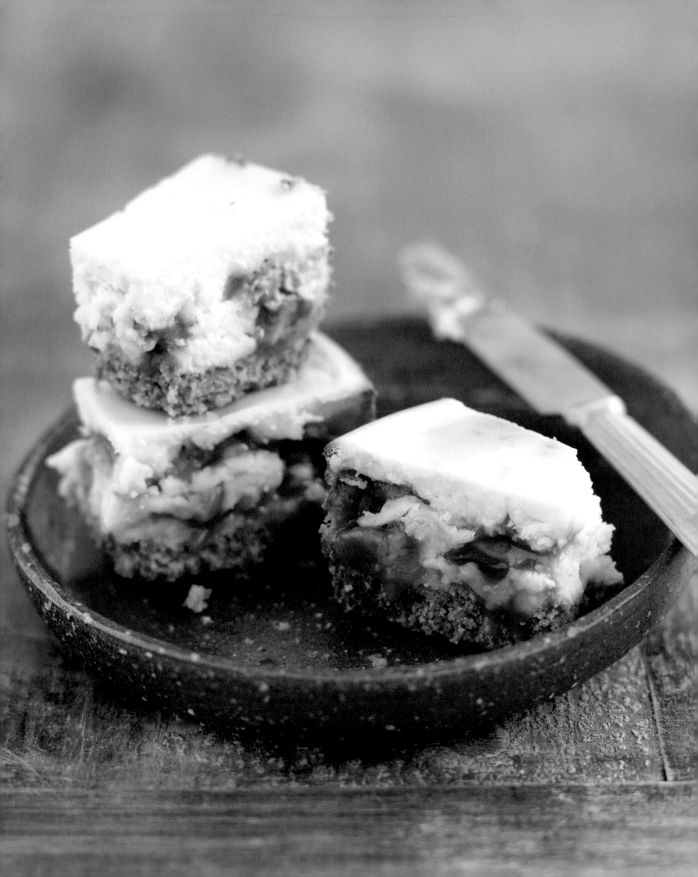

Baked Caramel Cheesecake

SERVES 14

You may wish to use the Simple Sweet Cookies (page 203) to make the crust for this cheesecake; otherwise, look for plain, gluten-free cookies in supermarkets and health-food stores. If you are lactose intolerant, only try a few bites.

7 ounces (200 g) Simple Sweet Cookies (page 203), or other gluten-free vanilla cookies

110 g unsalted butter, melted

Two 8-ounce packages (500 g) cream cheese, at room temperature

⅔ cup (150 g) superfine sugar

2 teaspoons vanilla extract

3 eggs

1 egg yolk

9 ounces (250 g) chewy caramels (gluten-free if following a gluten-free diet)

Confectioners' sugar, optional

1. Place the cookies in a food processor and pulse to make crumbs. Add the melted butter and pulse until well combined. Press the mixture into the bottom of the prepared pan, cover with plastic wrap, and refrigerate for 30 minutes.

2. Preheat the oven to 300°F (150°C) and grease an 8-inch (20 cm) springform pan.

3. Beat the cream cheese, sugar, and vanilla with an electric mixer until well combined. Add the eggs, one at a time, beating between additions, then add the egg yolk. Add the caramel pieces and stir well. Pour the mixture into the pan over the cookie crust and bake for 1 hour, or until just firm to touch.

4. Turn the oven off and leave the cheesecake in the oven with the oven door ajar for 4 hours, or until completely cool. (This prevents the cheesecake from cracking.) When cool, cover with plastic wrap and refrigerate for at least 2 hours before serving. Dust with confectioners' sugar, if desired.

PER SERVING (not including confectioners' sugar): 368 calories; 5.5 g protein; 25.3 g total fat; 15.7 g saturated fat; 31.1 g carbohydrates; 0.1 g fiber; 219 mg sodium

Polenta Cake with Lime and Strawberry Syrup

SERVES 12

The cornmeal and ground almonds give a pleasing grainy texture to this delectable cake. The lime and strawberry combination may seem a little unusual, but you'll love its delicious freshness. The cake may be served warm or at room temperature.

1. Preheat the oven to 320°F (160°C). Grease an 8-inch (20 cm) springform pan and line with parchment paper.

2. Beat the egg yolks, eggs, and sugar with an electric mixer until thick and pale. With a spoon, stir in the vanilla and lime zest. Combine the ground almonds, flour, cornmeal, and baking powder in a small bowl. Fold into the egg mixture. Add the melted butter and stir to combine.

3. Pour the mixture into the cake pan and bake for 45 to 55 minutes, until a toothpick inserted into the center comes out clean. Cover with foil halfway through baking to prevent over-browning. Remove from the oven and allow to cool in the pan for 10 minutes before transferring to a wire rack to cool completely.

4. To make the syrup, place the lime zest and juice, sugar, and ½ cup (125 ml) water in a medium saucepan, and stir over medium heat until the sugar has dissolved. Bring to a boil, then reduce the heat to low and add the strawberries. Simmer gently for 10 to 15 minutes, until the syrup has thickened and the strawberries have softened.

5. Cut the cake into slices and serve with a generous spoonful of the lime and strawberry syrup.

PER SERVING: 335 calories; 5.3 g protein; 18.6 g total fat; 7.9 g saturated fat; 38.2 g carbohydrates; 1.5 g fiber; 291 mg sodium

5 egg yolks

2 large eggs

1 cup (220 g) superfine sugar

2 teaspoons vanilla extract

Grated zest of 2 limes

1 cup (120 g) ground almonds

⅔ cup (90 g) fine rice flour

½ cup (65 g) coarse cornmeal

2 teaspoons baking powder (gluten-free if following a gluten-free diet)

10 tablespoons (150 g) unsalted butter, melted

LIME AND STRAWBERRY SYRUP

Grated zest and juice of 1 lime

½ cup (110 g) superfine sugar

8 ounces (200 g) strawberries, hulled and thickly sliced (about 1⅓ cups)

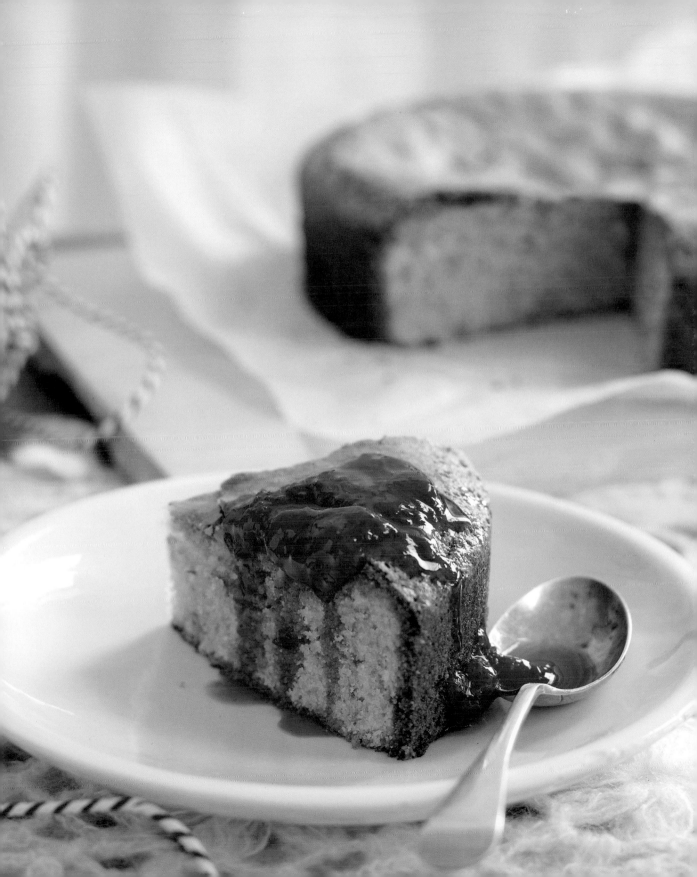

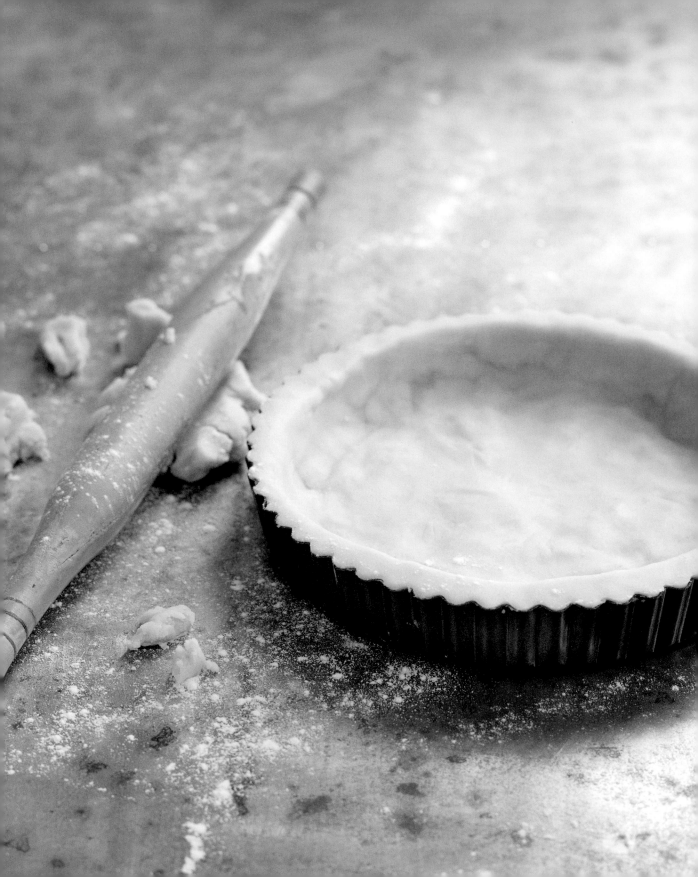

Citrus Tart

SERVES 10 TO 12

You will love the fresh flavors of this citrus tart. The trick to making the pastry is to add the water one tablespoon at a time—stop as soon as the desired consistency is achieved. Depending on the temperature in your kitchen, you may not need all the water specified. The amount of soy flour used in this recipe is minimal, so it will suit most people following the low-FODMAP diet. Assess your individual tolerance.

1. Preheat the oven to 350°F (170°C). Grease a 9-inch (23 cm) fluted tart dish with a removable bottom. To make the pastry, sift the rice flour, cornstarch, soy flour, and xanthan gum three times into a bowl (or mix with a whisk to ensure they are well combined). Transfer to a food processor. Add the sugar and butter and pulse until the mixture resembles fine crumbs. With the motor running, add the ice water, 1 tablespoon at a time, to form a soft dough. You may not need all the water. Turn out onto a cutting board dusted with cornstarch and knead until smooth. Cover with plastic wrap and refrigerate for 30 minutes.

2. Bring the dough to room temperature. Place between two sheets of parchment paper and roll out to ¼ inch (3 to 5 mm) thickness. Ease the pastry into the tart dish and trim the edges. Line the pastry with parchment paper, fill with baking beads or rice, and bake for 10 to 15 minutes, until lightly golden. Remove the parchment paper and beads (or rice).

3. Beat the sugar, lemon and orange juice, lemon and orange zest, and mascarpone in a small bowl. Add the eggs, one at a time, beating well between additions. Pour into the tart shell and bake for 1 hour, or until set and a toothpick inserted into the center comes out clean. Cool to room temperature and dust with confectioners' sugar. Serve with whipped cream, if desired.

PER SERVING (**one twelfth of recipe**): 318 calories; 3.9 g protein; 18.7 g total fat; 11.5 g saturated fat; 34.8 g carbohydrates; 0.5 g fiber; 38 mg sodium

PASTRY

1 cup (130 g) fine rice flour

½ cup (75 g) cornstarch

½ cup (45 g) soy flour

1 teaspoon xanthan gum

3 tablespoons superfine sugar

11 tablespoons (160 g) unsalted butter, chopped

⅓ to ½ cup (80 to 120 ml) ice water

FILLING

⅔ cup (150 g) superfine sugar

Juice from one lemon and one large ripe orange, ⅔ cup (150 ml) total

2 tablespoons lemon zest

1 tablespoon orange zest

5 ounces (150 g) mascarpone

3 eggs

Confectioners' sugar

Whipped cream, optional

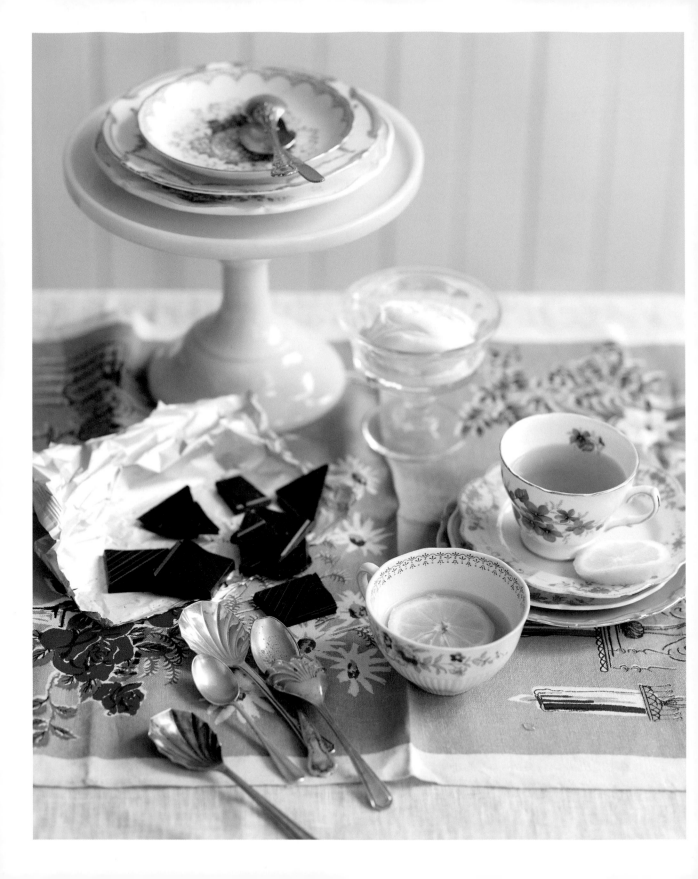

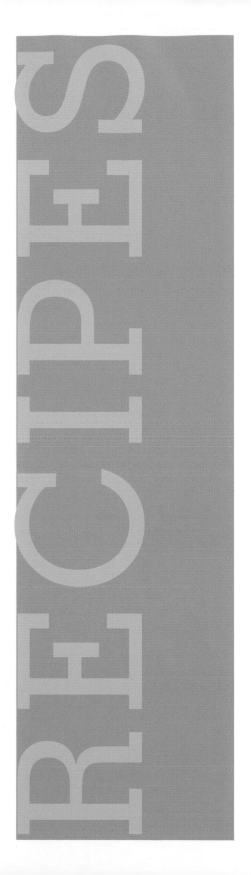

Puddings, Custards, and Ice Cream

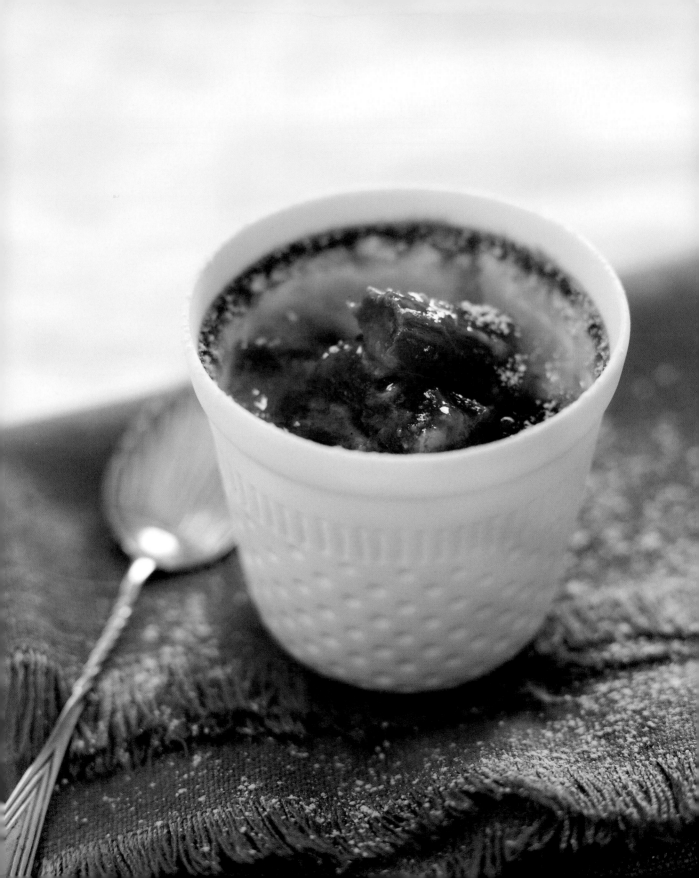

Dairy-Free Baked Rhubarb Custards

MAKES 6

This recipe suits those following the low-FODMAP diet, and is also dairy-free. The unique flavor of rhubarb tastes great in this delicious dessert, but 1 cup of stewed berries would also work well.

1. Preheat the oven to 350°F (180°C), and grease six 8-ounce (250 ml) ramekins.

2. Bring a large saucepan of water to a boil. Add the rhubarb and half of the superfine sugar, and cook over medium-high heat for 7 to 8 minutes, until the rhubarb has softened. Drain and discard the liquid. Spoon the rhubarb evenly into the ramekins. Place the ramekins in a large baking dish.

3. Combine the rice milk and vanilla in a small saucepan, and bring to a boil. Reduce the heat and simmer for 5 to 10 minutes, stirring regularly.

4. Whisk together the egg yolks and remaining superfine sugar in a heatproof bowl. Slowly pour in the warm milk, whisking constantly. Strain through a fine sieve into a clean saucepan. Cook over medium-low heat for 5 minutes, or until the custard simmers and starts to thicken.

5. Pour the custard over the rhubarb in the ramekins. Pour enough boiling water into the baking dish to come halfway up the sides of the ramekins. Bake on the lowest shelf of the oven for 30 to 35 minutes, until just firm. Remove the ramekins from the baking dish and set aside to cool for 5 minutes. Dust with confectioners' sugar and serve immediately.

PER SERVING: 255 calories; 4.1 g protein; 5.2 g total fat; 1.5 g saturated fat; 48 g carbohydrates; 2.4 g fiber; 84 mg sodium

5 rhubarb stalks, well washed and cut into 1-inch (2 cm) lengths

1 cup (220 g) superfine sugar

2 cups (500 ml) rice milk (gluten-free if following a gluten-free diet), or other milk if necessary

2 teaspoons vanilla bean paste, or the seeds of 1 vanilla bean or 2 teaspoon vanilla extract

6 egg yolks

Confectioners' sugar

Panna Cotta with Rosewater Cinnamon Syrup

MAKES 4

If you have ever tasted Turkish Delight, then you know the flavor of rosewater. Here, it is combined with cinnamon to make this light, creamy dessert something really special. If you are lactose intolerant, limit yourself to a half serving only.

1. Grease four 4-ounce (125 ml) dariole molds or tall ramekins.

2. Place the cream, milk, sugar, and vanilla bean paste in a small saucepan over low heat, and cook, stirring regularly, for 20 minutes, or until the mixture has thickened enough to coat the back of a spoon (do not allow it to boil). Remove from the heat.

3. Add 1 tablespoon of cold water to a small heatproof bowl and sprinkle the gelatin onto it while whisking with a fork. Set it aside for 5 minutes, or until it has begun to gel. Set the bowl in a larger bowl of boiling water and stir constantly until the gelatin has dissolved. Whisk into the custard. Pour the custard into a medium bowl.

4. Fill a large bowl with ice cubes. Set the custard on top of the ice-filled bowl and whisk every few minutes for about 10 minutes, or until thickened enough to coat the back of a wooden spoon. Pour into the molds and refrigerate for 2 to 3 hours.

5. Meanwhile, to make the syrup, combine the sugar, cinnamon, and ⅓ cup (80 ml) water in a small saucepan over low heat, and cook, stirring regularly, until the sugar has dissolved. Increase the heat to medium-high and bring to a boil. Reduce the heat and simmer gently for 5 to 7 minutes, until the liquid has reduced by half. Remove the pan from the heat, stir in the rosewater essence, and allow to cool to room temperature.

6. To serve, dip each mold in hot water for a few seconds, then turn out the custards onto plates. Drizzle the syrup over the top.

PER SERVING: 547 calories; 5.2 g protein; 38 g total fat; 24.4 g saturated fat; 50 g carbohydrates; 0 g fiber; 57 mg sodium

1⅔ cups (420 ml) light cream

½ cup (125 ml) low-fat milk, lactose-free milk, or suitable plant-based milk if necessary

½ cup (110 g) superfine sugar

2 teaspoons vanilla bean paste, or the seeds of 1 vanilla bean, or 2 teaspoons vanilla extract

2¼ teaspoons unflavored gelatin powder

ROSEWATER CINNAMON SYRUP

⅓ cup (75 g) superfine sugar

Two 1-inch (3 cm) pieces cinnamon stick

1½ teaspoons rose water

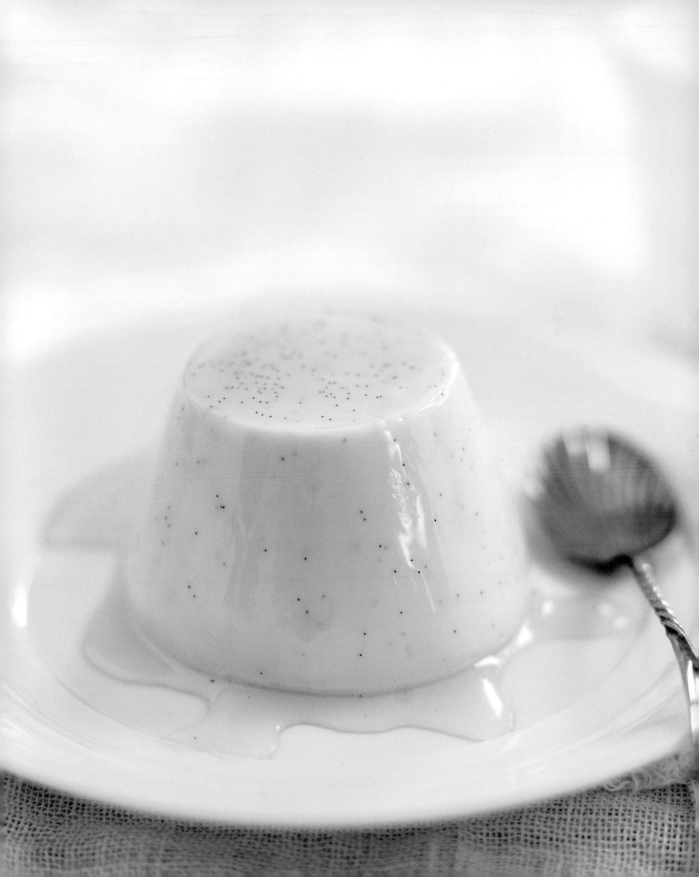

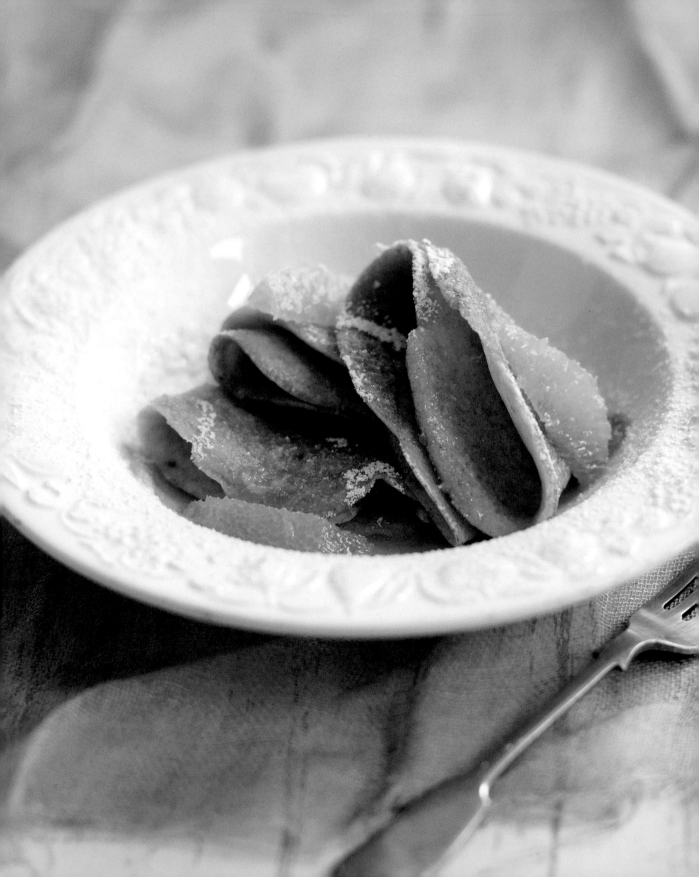

Crêpes Suzette

MAKES 8

This is the low-FODMAP version of what is probably the most famous crêpe dish ever. Traditionally, brandy is poured over the crêpes, then lit so the dessert is flaming when served, but I left this step out. The amount of soy flour used in the recipe is minimal, so it will suit most people following the low-FODMAP diet. Assess your individual tolerance—if necessary, replace the soy flour with tapioca flour.

1. Sift the rice flour, cornstarch, soy flour, and baking soda three times into a large bowl (or mix with a whisk so they are well combined). Make a well in the middle. Add the eggs, milk, sugar, and zest, and mix to form a smooth batter. Stir in the melted butter. Cover with plastic wrap and set aside for 20 minutes.

2. Heat a 7-inch (18 cm) nonstick skillet over medium heat and spray with cooking spray. Pour 2 to 3 tablespoons of batter into the pan and tilt to coat the entire surface. Cook until bubbles start to appear, then turn and cook the other side. Transfer to a plate and cover with foil to keep warm. Repeat with the remaining batter to make 8 crêpes in all, adding more cooking spray each time.

3. To make the sauce, combine the orange juice and zest, lemon zest, sugar, and liqueur in a small bowl. Melt the butter in the pan over low heat. Slowly add the juice mixture and heat gently.

4. Place one crêpe in the pan with the sauce and warm through. Fold it in half, and then in half again to make a wedge. Tilt the pan so the sauce flows away from the crêpe, then remove the crêpe and set aside on a warm plate. Cover with foil. Repeat with the remaining crêpes. When ready to serve, drizzle the crepes with any remaining sauce. Serve with the orange segments, dusted with confectioners' sugar if desired.

PER SERVING: 297 calories; 6.2 g protein; 15.4 g total fat; 8.9 g saturated fat; 34 g carbohydrates; 0.8 g fiber; 147 mg sodium

¾ cup (130 g) rice flour

½ cup (75 g) cornstarch

⅓ cup (30 g) soy flour

¾ teaspoon baking soda

2 eggs, lightly beaten

2 cups (500 ml) low-fat milk, lactose-free milk, or suitable plant-based milk

2 tablespoons superfine sugar

1 tablespoon grated orange zest

3 tablespoons (40 g) butter, melted

Cooking spray

SUZETTE SAUCE

1 cup (250 ml) orange juice

Grated zest of 2 oranges

Grated zest of 1 small lemon

1 teaspoon superfine sugar, or more to taste

¼ cup (60 ml) Grand Marnier or Cointreau, or an additional ¼ cup (60 ml) orange juice

6 tablespoons (80 g) butter

Orange segments

Confectioners' sugar, optional

Caramel Banana Tapioca Puddings

MAKES 6

Cooked tapioca is the base for these soft, creamy puddings. People with lactose intolerance should use lactose-free milk.

1. Place the milk, vanilla, and ¼ cup (60 g) of the brown sugar in a medium saucepan, and bring to a boil over medium-high heat, stirring well. Reduce the heat to low and stir in the pearl tapioca. Simmer gently, stirring regularly, for 30 to 35 minutes, until the tapioca is soft and resembles translucent jelly-like balls. Set aside to cool for 5 to 10 minutes.

2. In a large bowl, mix the mashed banana with half of the remaining brown sugar. Stir in the cooked tapioca. Pour the mixture evenly into six 4-ounce (125 ml) ramekins. Sprinkle the tops with the rest of the brown sugar and refrigerate for 3 to 4 hours, until set.

PER SERVING: 228 calories; 6.8 g protein; 2.2 g total fat; 1.4 g saturated fat; 46 g carbohydrates; 0.6 g fiber; 72 mg sodium

4 cups (1 liter) low-fat milk, lactose-free milk, or suitable plant-based milk

2 teaspoons vanilla extract

¼ cup (60 g) plus ⅓ cup (75 g) brown sugar

⅓ cup (65 g) pearl tapioca or sago

2 ripe bananas, mashed with a fork

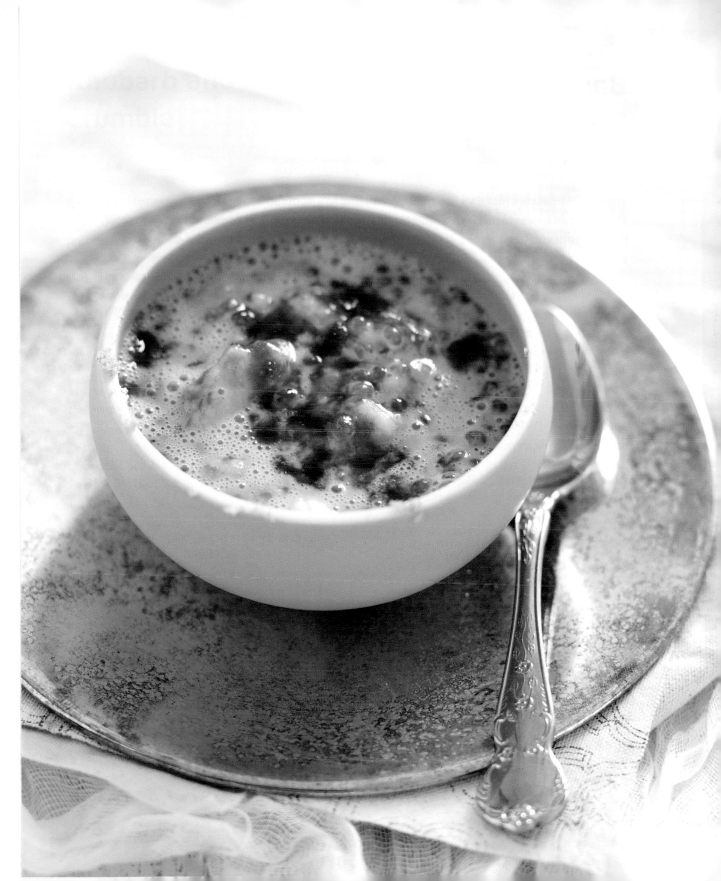

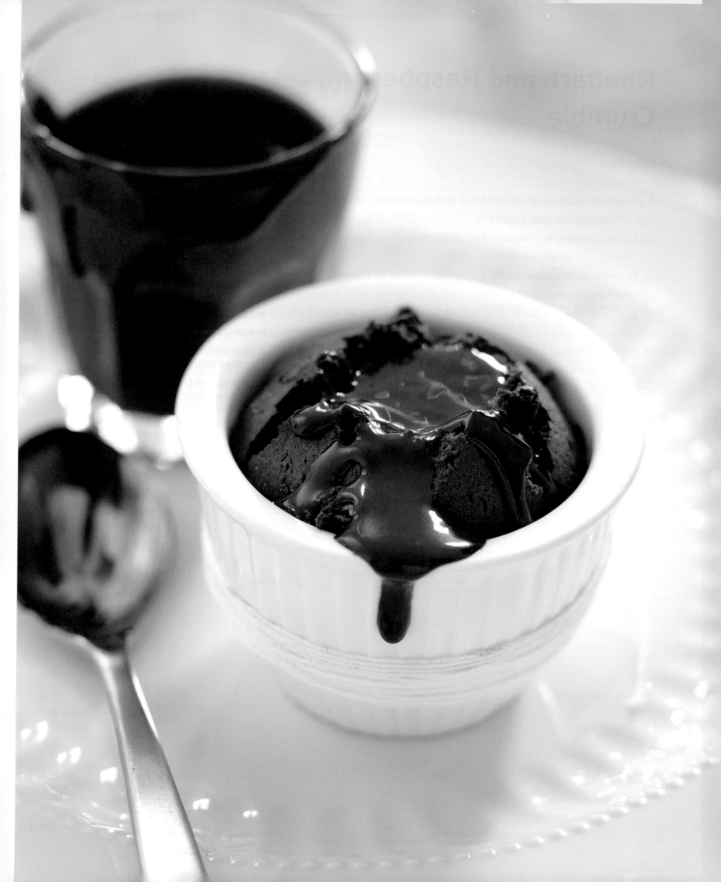

Gooey Chocolate Puddings

MAKES 8

If you don't have ceramic ramekins, you can use a large Texas muffin pan for these decadent puddings. For a final flourish, serve them with fresh strawberries and whipped cream.

1. Preheat the oven to 350°F (180°C). Grease eight 4-ounce (175 ml) ramekins.

2. Place the chocolate and butter in a small saucepan and stir over low heat for 5 minutes, or until smooth and completely melted. Allow to cool for 5 minutes. Beat the eggs, egg yolks, and brown sugar with an electric mixer for 5 to 10 minutes, until doubled in volume. With a spoon, fold in the cooled chocolate. Sprinkle the rice flour over the mixture and gently fold in.

3. Spoon the batter into the ramekins. Place on a baking sheet and bake for 7 to 10 minutes, until just firm to touch.

4. Meanwhile, to make the sauce, place the chocolate and cream in a small saucepan over medium-low heat. Stir until the chocolate has melted and the sauce is smooth and well combined. Stir in the confectioners' sugar.

5. Turn out the puddings onto individual plates, or serve in the ramekins. Drizzle with the chocolate sauce and serve warm.

PER SERVING: 514 calories, 6.7 g protein; 36.2 g total fat; 21.6 g saturated fat; 43.0 g carbohydrates; 0.5 g fiber; 68 mg sodium

7 ounces (200 g) dark chocolate

10 tablespoons (150 g) unsalted butter, chopped

4 eggs, at room temperature

4 egg yolks, at room temperature

½ cup (110 g) brown sugar

¼ cup (40 g) fine rice flour

CHOCOLATE SAUCE

3½ ounces (100 g) dark chocolate

½ cup (125 ml) light whipping cream

1½ tablespoons confectioners' sugar

Cinnamon Chili Chocolate Brûlées

MAKES 6

Here's an interesting combination: rich creamy chocolate pots with a surprise chili kick. If you prefer a gentler nudge of chili, reduce the quantity to just a pinch. If you have access to couverture chocolate (a gourmet variety with more cocoa butter than other kinds), use that in this recipe. Otherwise, choose any high-quality dark chocolate. Note that you need to start preparing this dish the day before serving. Limit yourself to a half serving if you are lactose intolerant.

2½ cups (600 ml) light whipping cream

4 ounces (125 g) dark chocolate

2 teaspoons ground cinnamon

¼ teaspoon chili powder

6 egg yolks

½ cup (110 g) superfine sugar

1. Preheat the oven to 300°F (150°C). Place six 4-ounce (125 ml) ramekins in a baking dish.

2. Place the cream, chocolate, cinnamon, and chili powder in a medium saucepan, and stir over medium heat until smooth and the chocolate has melted. Remove from the heat and cool to room temperature.

3. Beat the egg yolks and ⅓ cup (75 g) of the sugar with an electric mixer until pale and creamy. Add the cooled chocolate mixture and beat until well combined. Divide the mixture among the ramekins. Pour enough boiling water into the baking dish to come halfway up the sides of the ramekins. Bake on the lowest shelf of the oven for 45 to 50 minutes, until firm around the edges. Remove the ramekins from the baking dish and let cool to room temperature (about one hour). Cover with plastic wrap and refrigerate for 8 hours or overnight to set.

4. Sprinkle the remaining sugar over the brûlées and broil until the sugar bubbles and caramelizes, about 3 to 5 minutes. (Alternatively, use a kitchen blowtorch to do this.) Set aside for 5 minutes before serving.

PER SERVING: 553 calories; 5.6 g protein; 45.7 g total fat; 27.9 g saturated fat; 33.2 g carbohydrates; 0.3 g fiber; 56 mg sodium

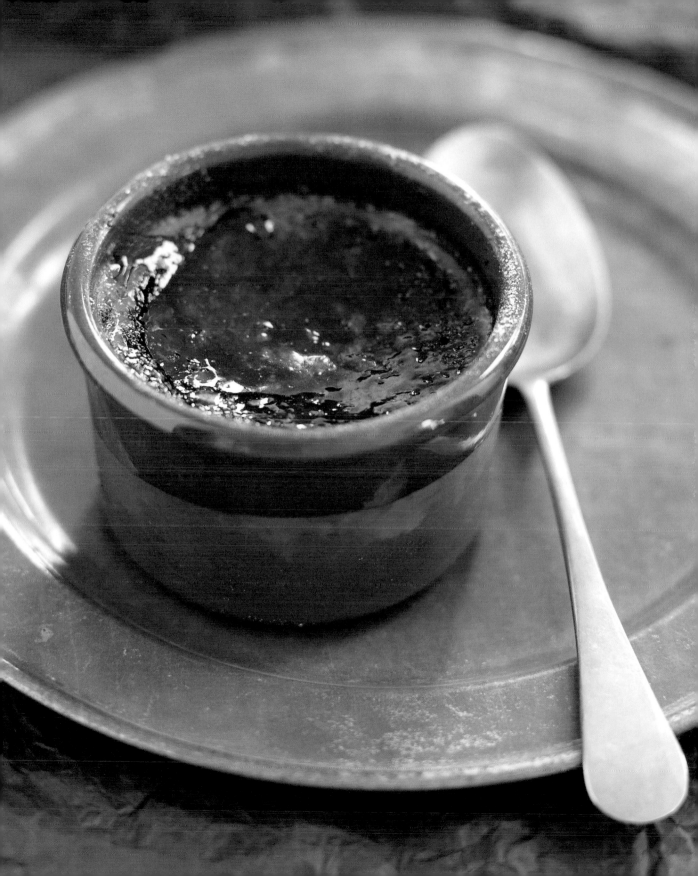

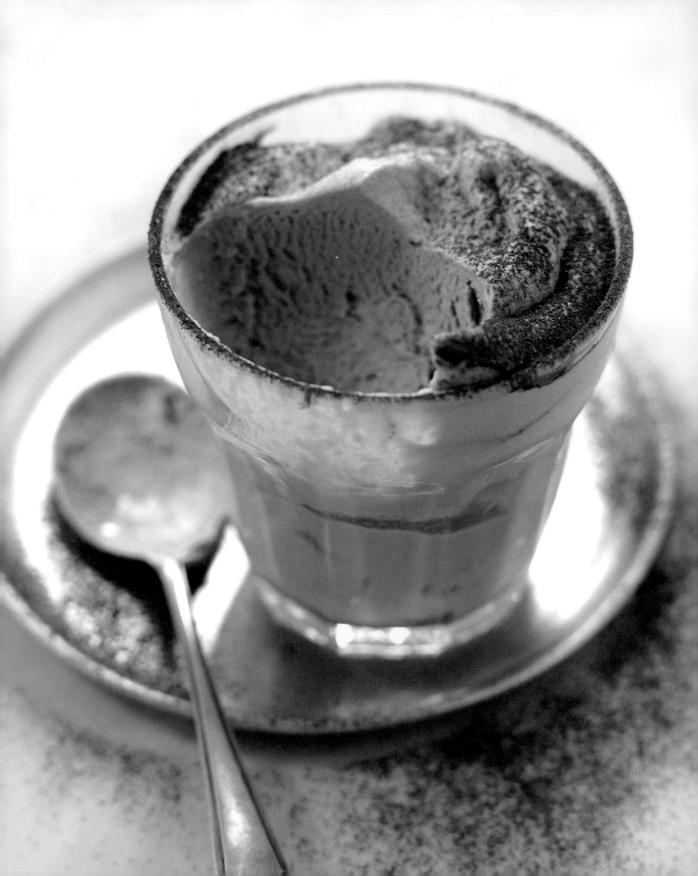

Frozen Cappuccino

SERVES 6 TO 8

This ice cream recipe makes enough for six good-size portions, but I often use it to make eight smaller servings—there is still enough to ensure everyone gets a satisfying share! If you are lactose intolerant, limit yourself to a half-serving.

1. Beat the egg whites and half of the sugar until stiff glossy peaks form.

2. Combine the coffee, remaining sugar, and ⅓ cup (80 ml) water in a small saucepan and stir over medium-high heat until the mixture is bubbling and syrupy. If you have a sugar thermometer, the syrup should be heated to 250°F (120°C).

3. Slowly pour the coffee syrup into the egg whites and beat until well combined. Cover with plastic wrap and refrigerate until completely chilled.

4. Beat the cream with an electric mixer until firm peaks form. Gently fold in the mascarpone with a spoon. Fold in the cold coffee mixture until well combined. Pour into six or eight dessert bowls, glasses, or small coffee cups, and freeze for 4 hours. Take out of the freezer 5 minutes before serving. Dust with cocoa powder, if desired.

PER SERVING (one eighth of recipe): 249 calories; 2.7 g protein; 15.5 g total fat; 10.1 g saturated fat; 26.6 g carbohydrates; 0.1 g fiber; 46 mg sodium

4 egg whites

¾ cup plus 2 tablespoons (200 g) superfine sugar

2 tablespoons instant coffee

⅔ cup (170 ml) light whipping cream

¾ cup (6 ounces/180 g) mascarpone, or the same amount of cream cheese plus 1 teaspoon vanilla extract

Cocoa powder, optional

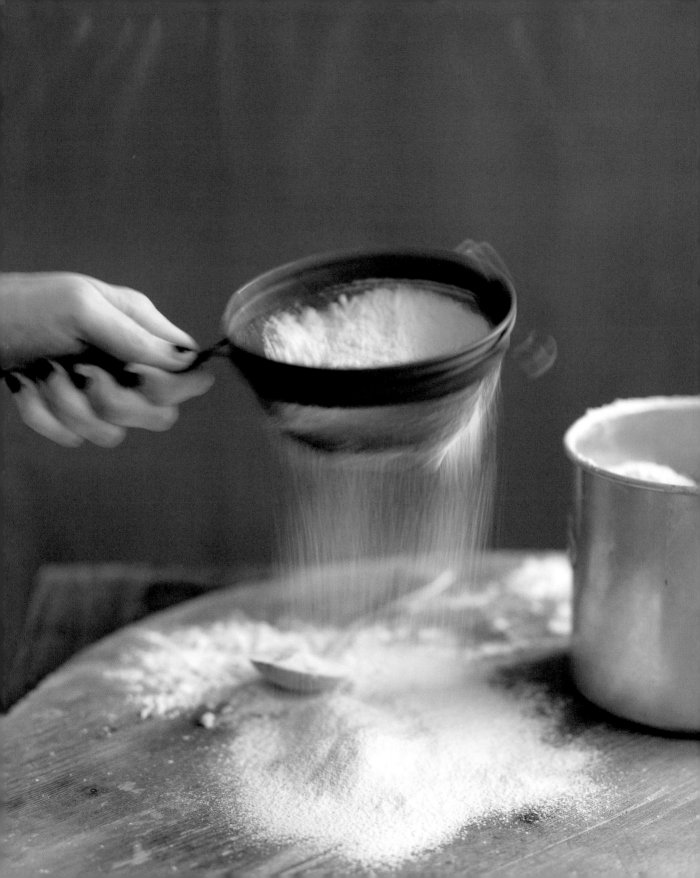

Baking powder

Baking powder is a leavener (raising agent). Not all baking powders are gluten-free—always check the label before buying. A simple recipe for baking powder is 1 teaspoon cream of tartar and ½ teaspoon baking soda. This can be added to 1 cup of a wheat-free flour blend to make it "self-rising."

Buckwheat

Despite its name, buckwheat is not related to wheat at all—it is actually a member of the rhubarb family. It has a strong nutty flavor and is often made into flour and used in recipes such as pancakes.

Cornmeal

Cornmeal can be cooked into polenta or used in rustic gluten-free breads and cakes. It is available in three textures: fine, medium, and coarse. For added nutrition, it is worth seeking out stone-ground cornmeal, which retains more of the corn's hull and germ. Cornmeal can be found at any grocery store, but the stone-ground variety may only be available at specialty stores or online.

Cornstarch

Cornstarch is a gluten-free ingredient made from corn. In some countries (such as Australia and New Zealand) flour made from wheat can be called cornstarch, but in the United States this should not be the case. It has little taste, is low in protein, and makes an excellent addition to a wheat-free flour blend. It is perfect for thickening sauces.

Potato flour

Made from potato starch, potato flour is virtually tasteless. It can be used to thicken sweet and savory sauces; however, the sauce will become a little "stretchy" or gel-like. It is great in a wheat-free flour blend, especially for cakes and muffins, and makes a good substitute for tapioca flour and arrowroot. It is available in grocery stores.

Quinoa

Pronounced "keen-wah," quinoa can be used in a variety of ways, including being made into pasta and flour. The whole grain can be cooked like rice and used as a base for salads or side dishes. It has a slightly bitter taste. It is available from grocery and health-food stores.

Rice flour

White rice flour is the main component in many wheat-free flour blends and is an essential addition to any wheat-free pantry. The texture ranges from fine to gritty. Fine rice flour is preferable and is readily available in Asian grocery stores. Superfine is even better and is available online. It has a neutral taste and can be used as a thickener for sauces and gravies. Brown rice flour is also available and can be used in wheat-free baking to increase the fiber content.

Soy flour

Soy flour is a high-protein flour made from soybeans. It can have a strong, sometimes bitter flavor. This bitterness decreases with cooking, but it is better to purchase debittered soy flour if possible. Soy flour is best used as a small part of a wheat-free flour blend. It is available from health-food stores.

Superfine sugar

Superfine sugar, sometimes known as caster sugar, is finer than regular granulated sugar, so it dissolves faster. It is worth seeking out for the recipes in this book that call for it, because substituting granulated sugar may result in a gritty texture. Many grocery stores carry superfine sugar, but you can also make it at home by processing granulated sugar in a food processor.

Tapioca flour

Tapioca flour is made from the dried starch of the cassava root. It has little flavor, is low in protein, and is a useful addition to a wheat-free flour blend. It can be used to thicken sweet and savory sauces, but the sauce will become a little "stretchy" and gel-like. It is a good substitute for potato flour and arrow-root. It is available in Asian grocery stores and some health-food stores.

Xanthan gum

Xanthan gum is a vegetable gum used in baked goods to help provide elasticity and keep them moist. It is a cream-colored powder made from the ground, dried cell coat of a laboratory-grown microorganism called *Xanthomonas campestris*. It is the most common vegetable gum used in wheat-free cooking, though guar gum or cellulose gum (CMC) can be used instead. It is available from health-food stores.

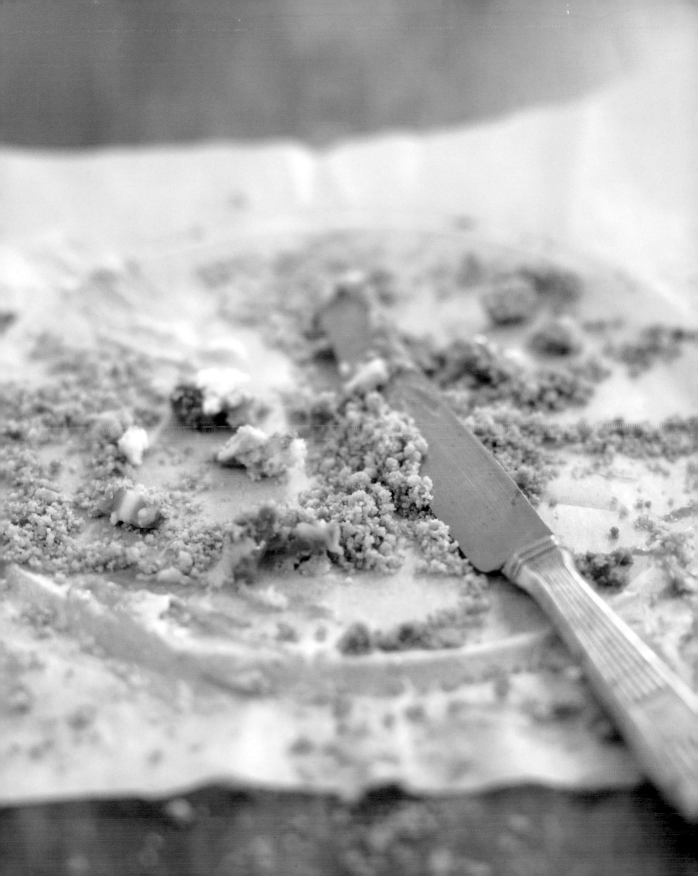

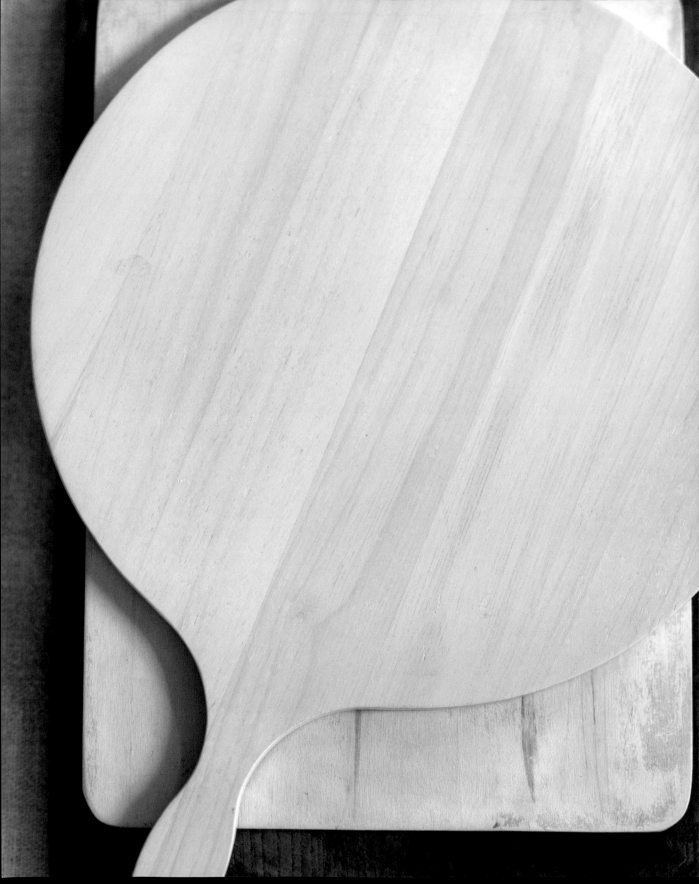

THIS BOOK cannot possibly cover all topics of relevance to the low-FODMAP diet. In order to follow the low-FODMAP diet more easily, it is essential to be equipped with books like this one, but here are some other sources that might help you with following the diet, finding a dietitian, and learning about digestion.

Our book's website

www.thelowfodmapdiet.com

Our book's website offers additional information on various topics, as indicated throughout the book.

Registered Dietitians

Several times in this book, we recommend seeking the advice of a registered dietitian. Ask your gastroenterologist or GP about dietitians with expertise in the low-FODMAP diet. If they cannot help, you could try the following.

For readers in the United States: The Academy of Nutrition and Dietetics, "Find a Registered Dietitian"

www.eatright.org/programs/rdfinder

Search for "Digestive Disorders" and/or "Food Allergies/Food Intolerance."

For readers in Canada: Dietitians of Canada, "Find a Dietitian"

www.dietitians.ca/Find-a-Dietitian.aspx.

Search by keyword "irritable bowel," "digestive disorders," "celiac disease," etc.

Additional Resources For Digestive Disorders

American College of Gastroenterology
www.acg.gi.org

American Dietetic Association
www.eatright.org

Canadian Digestive Health Foundation
www.cdhf.ca

National Digestive Diseases Information Clearinghouse
www.digestive.niddk.nih.gov

International Foundation for Functional Gastrointestinal Disorders
www.iffgd.org

Rome III Diagnostic Questionnaires
www.romecriteria.org/questionnaires

Irritable Bowel Syndrome Self Help and Support Group

www.ibsgroup.org

National Foundation for Celiac Awareness

www.celiaccentral.org

Crohn's and Colitis Foundation of America

www.ccfa.org

Food Diary

Copy the food diary that follows (or download it from this book's website) and use it to keep track of your daily FODMAP intake. You will find it very useful not only to work out which foods cause your symptoms to flare up, but also if you decide at any stage to consult a registered dietitian.

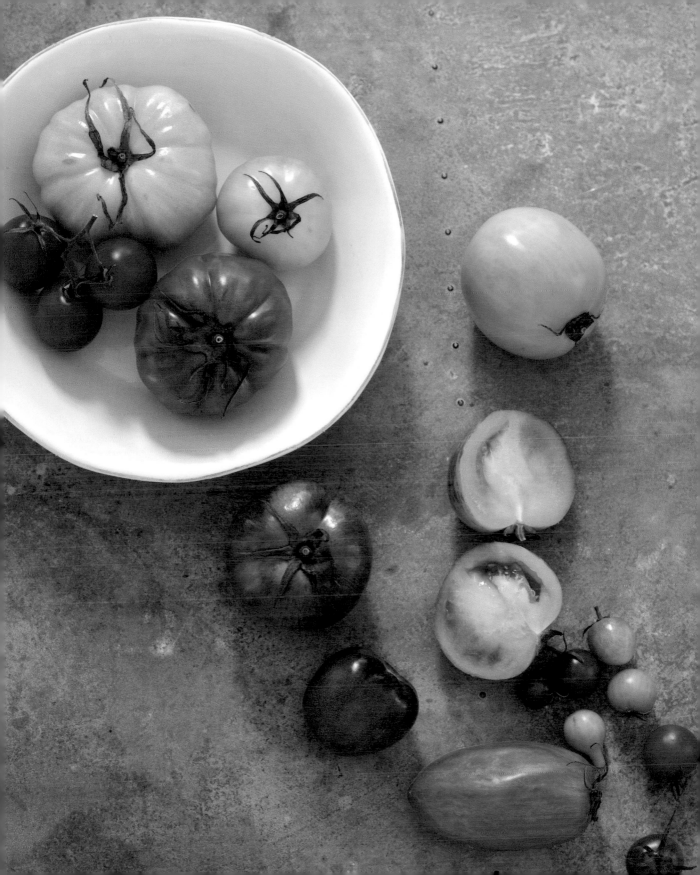

YOUR FOOD DIARY

WEEK _____

DAY	BREAKFAST	MIDMORNING SNACK	LUNCH

AFTERNOON SNACK	DINNER	EVENING SNACK	SYMPTOMS

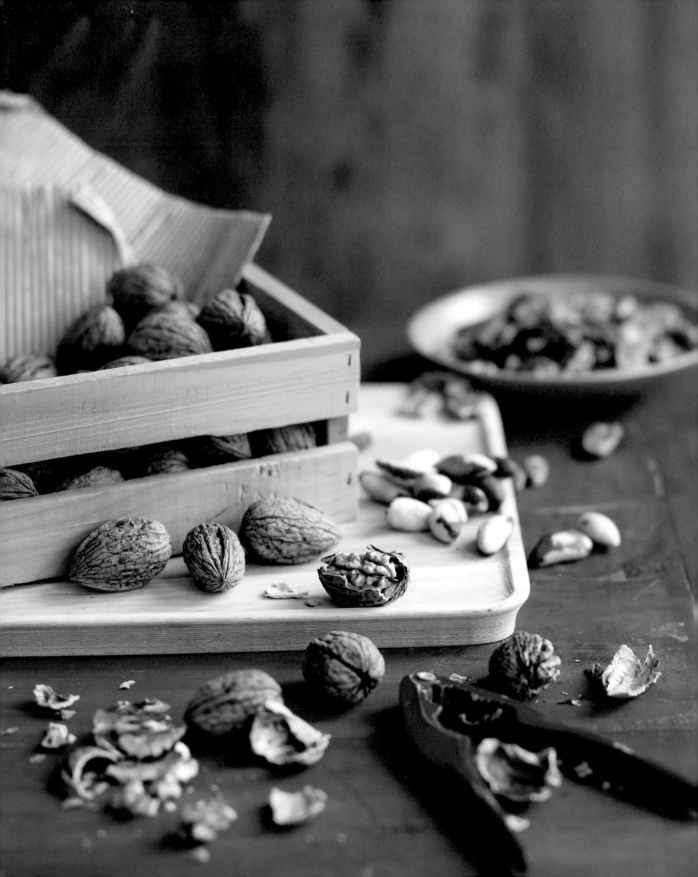

Review articles

ON FODMAPS, THE LOW-FODMAP DIET, AND BREATH HYDROGEN TESTING

Barrett, Jacqueline S., and Peter R. Gibson. "Fructose and Lactose Testing." *Australian Family Physician* 41, no. 5 (2012): 293–96.

Gibson, Peter R., E. Newnham, Jacqueline S. Barrett, Susan J. Shepherd, and Jane G. Muir. "Fructose Malabsorption and the Bigger Picture." *Alimentary Pharmacology and Therapeutics* 25, no.4 (2007): 349–63

Gibson, Peter R., and Susan J. Shepherd. "Evidence-Based Dietary Management of Functional Gastrointestinal Symptoms: The FODMAP Approach." *Journal of Gastroenterology and Hepatology* 25, no. 2 (2009): 252–58.

Gibson, Peter R., and Susan J. Shepherd. "Food Choice as a Key Management Strategy for Functional Gastrointestinal Symptoms." *The American Journal of Gastroenterology* 107, no. 5 (2012): 657–66.

Shepherd, Susan J., Miranda C. E. Lomer, and Peter R. Gibson. "Short-Chain Carbohydrates and Functional Gastrointestinal Disorders." *The American Journal of Gastroenterology* 108, no. 5 (2013): 707–17.

Original research papers

ON THE LOW-FODMAP DIET IN GENERAL AND FOR PEOPLE WITH IRRITABLE BOWEL SYNDROME

Barrett, Jacqueline S., Richard B. Gearry, Jane G. Muir, Peter M. Irving, Rosemary Rose, Ourania Rosella, M. L. Haines, Susan J. Shepherd, and Peter R. Gibson. "Dietary Poorly Absorbed, Short-Chain Carbohydrates Increase Delivery of Water and Fermentable Substrates to the Proximal Colon." *Alimentary Pharmacology and Therapeutics* 31, no. 8 (2010): 874–82.

Ong, Derrick K., Shaylyn B. Mitchell, Jacqueline S. Barrett, Sue J. Shepherd, Peter M. Irving, Jessica R. Biesiekierski, Stuart Smith, Peter R. Gibson, and Jane G. Muir. "Manipulation of Dietary Short Chain Carbohydrates Alters the Pattern of Gas Production and Genesis of Symptoms in Irritable Bowel Syndrome." *Journal of Gastroenterology and Hepatology* 25, no. 8 (2010): 1366–73.

Shepherd, Susan J., Francis C. Parker, Jane G. Muir, and Peter R. Gibson. "Dietary Triggers of Abdominal Symptoms in Patients With Irritable Bowel Syndrome: Randomized Placebo-Controlled Evidence." *Clinical Gastroenterology and Hepatology* 6, no. 7 (2008): 765–71.

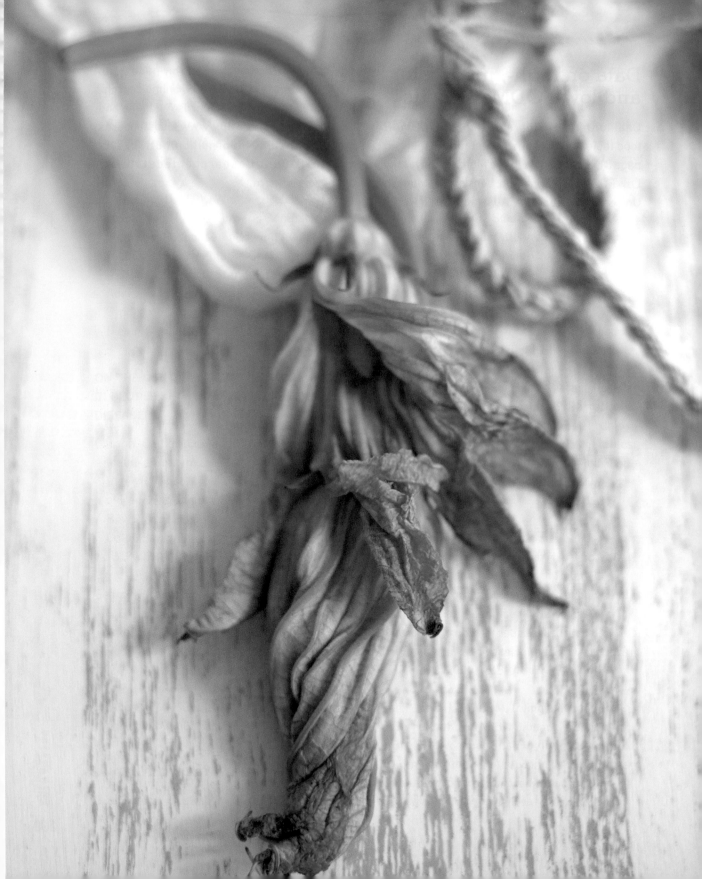

ACKNOWLEDGMENTS

IT IS A PLEASURABLE but difficult task to duly acknowledge all of the wonderful people who have supported us on this great journey to introduce our FODMAP concept to the international stage.

Thanks first to our families and friends. Over many years, you have listened to stories of our progress and provided enthusiastic support for each of our achievements. We thank you for sharing it all and know this is as much a celebration for you as it is for us.

To the team at the Department of Gastroenterology, Alfred Hospital (formerly at Eastern Health Clinical School), Monash University: Your hard work and diligence in research excellence have helped further develop and realize FODMAP concepts. Your efforts are greatly appreciated and it is a privilege to work with you. Thanks to the dietitians at Shepherd Works, who have helped support the growth of FODMAP research by applying it to so many patients. To all our colleagues who are clinicians and clinical researchers in the Department of Gastroenterology and Hepatology at Eastern Health/Box Hill Hospital: Thank you for believing in us. We also thank many medical colleagues outside Eastern Health who have embraced and supported the concepts. To our professional associations, the Dietitian's Association of Australia and the Gastroenterological Society of Australia, we so appreciate your enthusiastic acknowledgment of this innovative therapy. And sincere gratitude to our patients, who provide us with such a sense of purpose, motivating us to do our very best at all times. Thanks also to inspirational foodie friends Jo Richardson, Tobie Puttock, Peta Gray, and Spencer Clements.

We are indebted to the wonderful team at Penguin Australia for having confidence in the FODMAP concept, and for allowing us to describe it so comprehensively to help improve the quality of life of so many. Thanks to Julie Gibbs and Ingrid Ohlsson for your belief, and Rachel Carter and Nicola Young for editorial excellence. Thanks to photographer Mark O'Meara, food stylist Sarah O'Brien, and home economist Tracey Meharg for the mouthwatering photographs, and to Megan Pigott for overseeing the shoot. Thanks also to Elissa Webb for her sensational design.

We would also like to thank the team at The Experiment, who have worked tirelessly to make this book perfectly pitched to the North American public. Thanks to Matthew Lore, the publisher, who sought our bestselling book from Australia to launch in the US. Enormous thanks to Molly Cavanaugh for your hours and hours dedicated to the editing required to "Americanize" our book. You have been a delight to work with. We also appreciate Cara Bedick, Lukas Volger, and Maryanne Bannon for their editorial assistance. Thanks to Jack Palmer and Sarah Schneider for marketing and promotion. Also, thanks to Katherine Kelly, dietitian, for preparing the nutritional analyses of all the recipes.

To the friends, colleagues, and acquaintances who have not been specifically mentioned, thank you for your very special role in our lives.

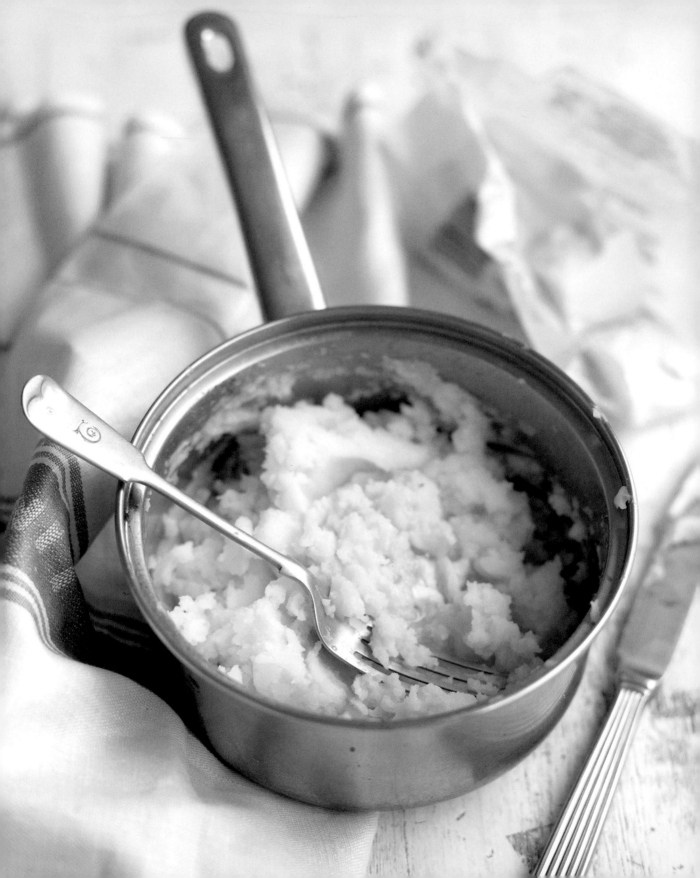

INDEX

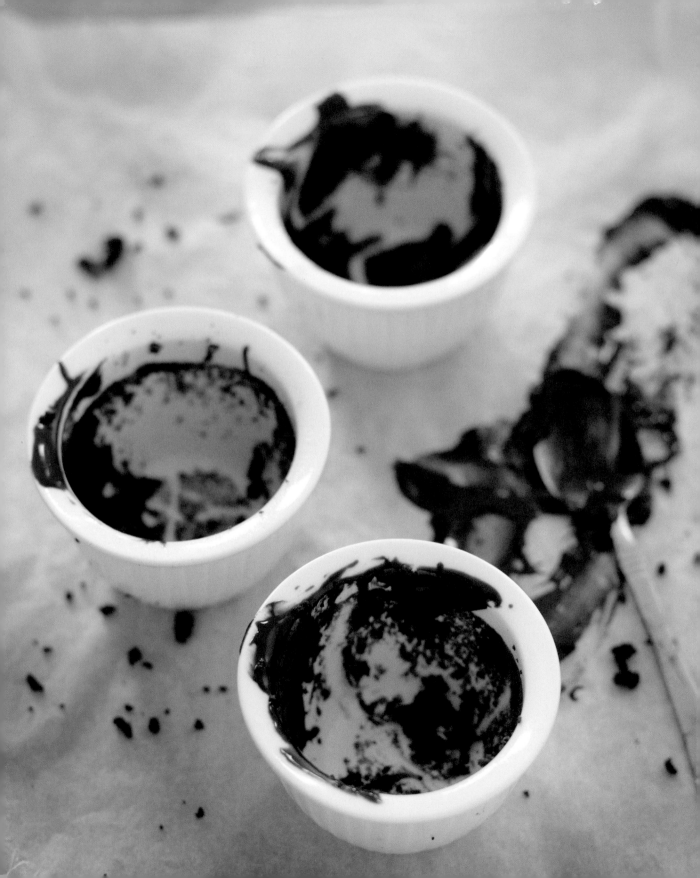

SUE SHEPHERD, PhD, an Advanced Accredited Practicing Dietitian and Accredited Nutritionist, specializes in the treatment of dietary intolerances. She has a Bachelor of Applied Science in Health Promotion, a Masters in Nutrition and Dietetics, and a PhD for her research into the low-FODMAP diet, celiac disease, and irritable bowel syndrome. Sue, who has celiac disease herself, lives and breathes gluten-free and low-FODMAP. For creating the low-FODMAP diet, a world-first scientifically proven diet for people with IBS, she was awarded the Telstra Australian Businesswoman of the year, State Finalist (Victoria) award and the Gastroenterological Society of Australia's Young Investigator Award. She is the author of numerous peer-reviewed international medical journal publications, and is an invited speaker at international medical conferences as she is recognized internationally as an expert dietitian in the field of IBS and celiac disease. She has authored ten cookbooks for people with celiac disease, FODMAP intolerance, and irritable bowel syndrome, and runs Australia's largest dietitian private practice specializing in gastrointestinal nutrition called Shepherd Works (www.shepherd works.com.au), where Sue and her team of expert dietitians treat people with these conditions, including overseas consultations via Skype. She is the consultant dietitian on medical international advisory committees for gastrointestinal conditions, is on the editorial committee for Australia's leading health magazine, *Healthy Food Guide*, regularly consults to the media, and was the resident dietitian on a national television program. Sue is now a Senior Lecturer and Senior Researcher at the Department of Dietetics and Human Nutrition at La Trobe University in Melbourne, Australia, where she heads this department's research into FODMAPs. She also has a line of low-FODMAP food products.

PETER GIBSON, MD, is Professor of Gastroenterology, Monash University and Director of the Department of Gastroenterology at the Alfred Hospital, Melbourne. He was formerly Professor of Medicine and Head of the Eastern Health Clinical School and Executive Clinical Director of Specialty Medicine and Director of Gastroenterology and Hepatology for Eastern Health. After completing his medical degree with first-class honors, he pursued training in gastroenterology at Melbourne's Alfred Hospital and the John Radcliffe Hospital in Oxford, UK. In 1985 he was awarded an MD for his work on immunology and the bowel. After three years as a Research Fellow at the Australian National University, he joined the Department of Medicine at the University of Melbourne and the Royal Melbourne Hospital, where he was later Deputy Director of Gastroenterology. In 2001 he moved to Box Hill Hospital and in 2011 to the Alfred Hospital. A past president of the Gastroenterological Society of Australia, Peter has a long-standing interest in the influence of diet on bowel health. He has an international reputation as both a physician and researcher for such conditions as inflammatory bowel disease, celiac disease, and irritable bowel syndrome. He was recently awarded the Distinguished Research Prize by the Gastroenterological Society of Australia. Peter now leads a Monash University research team of dietitians, scientists, and clinicians who are continuing to refine and extend our knowledge of the low-FODMAP diet.